Praise for *Chakra Empowerment*

"Lisa has provided a much-needed resource for w
trauma survivors who wish to include self-guided e.
their healing process. Every survivor is unique, and finding a variety of trauma-
sensitive resources to draw upon is essential. With this gentle and inclusive
guide, Lisa has added richly to these resources."

—Molly Boeder Harris, founder and
executive director of the Breathe Network

"Lisa offers us a way to work with our mind and body holistically through
our energy anatomy. These guided exercises can be used in combination with
other healing modalities or on their own, allowing us each to tailor them
to our individual needs. Women of all backgrounds will find something of
value in these tools."

—Madisyn Taylor, cofounder of *DailyOM* and author of
Unmedicated: The Four Pillars of Natural Wellness

"Lisa Erickson has created an insight-filled, empowering, and accessible guide
to learning about feminine energetics. Her systematic, step-by-step approach
effectively guides the reader toward sensing, healing, and wisely utilizing her
own energetic system. What a gift!"

—Robin King, author of *Joy's Edge: Transforming Your Life
Through Mindfulness, Wisdom, and Compassion*

"Lisa Erickson takes women on a masterful journey to getting unstuck so
we can evolve to the next level of our being. Filled with explanations, affirmations, visualization exercises, and other creative ways to move blocked
energy throughout our chakras, this book is a must-read for all of us."

—Meryl Davids Landau, author of *Warrior Won*

"I am extremely grateful to Lisa Erickson for exploring the distinctly female
energetics within the chakra system to create tools for women to heal from
abusive power. Using the beautifully constructed visualizations, affirmations,
and exercises provided, women who read this book will be able to move forward empowered with their inherent strength and wisdom renewed."

—Ra··a Chopra, author of *The Chakra Energy Diet: The Right Food,
Relaxation, Yoga & Exercise to Look and Feel Your Best*

"Not only are these chakra empowerments authentic and powerful, they are refreshingly pragmatic. I think the case studies, in particular, make these empowerments very accessible. Reading other women's stories and seeing how the empowerments are employed and the benefit they provided gives you a real understanding of how they can shift your entire way of being in the world."

—Sara Weston, author of *How to Be Happy Now: Even If Things Aren't Going Your Way*

Chakra
Empowerment
FOR Women

About the Author

Lisa Erickson is a chakra-based energy worker, writer, and teacher specializing in women's energetics and sexual trauma healing. She has meditated for over thirty years, taught for fifteen, and is certified in both mindfulness meditation instruction and trauma sensitivity. Lisa is a member of the International Association of Meditation Instructors, the American Holistic Health Association, and the Energy Medicine Practitioners Association. She is also the creator of a popular *DailyOM* course called *Awakening Your Feminine Chakras*. Visit her online at www.ChakraEmpowermentForWomen.com.

To Write to the Author

If you wish to contact the author or would like more information about this book, please write to the author in care of Llewellyn Worldwide Ltd. and we will forward your request. Both the author and publisher appreciate hearing from you and learning of your enjoyment of this book and how it has helped you. Llewellyn Worldwide Ltd. cannot guarantee that every letter written to the author can be answered, but all will be forwarded. Please write to:

Lisa Erickson
℅ Llewellyn Worldwide
2143 Wooddale Drive
Woodbury, MN 55125-2989

Please enclose a self-addressed stamped envelope for reply,
or $1.00 to cover costs. If outside the U.S.A., enclose
an international postal reply coupon.

Many of Llewellyn's authors have websites with additional
information and resources. For more information,
please visit our website at http://www.llewellyn.com

FOREWORD BY CYNDI DALE

LISA ERICKSON

SELF-GUIDED TECHNIQUES FOR
HEALING TRAUMA, OWNING YOUR POWER
& FINDING OVERALL WELLNESS

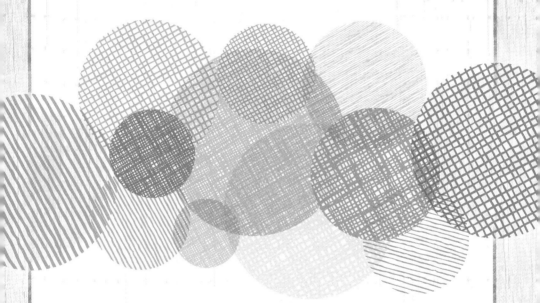

Chakra
Empowerment
FOR Women

LLEWELLYN PUBLICATIONS
WOODBURY, MINNESOTA

First Edition
First Printing, 2019

Book design by Samantha Penn
Cover design by Shira Atakpu
Editing by Laura Kurtz
Illustrations by Mary Ann Zapalac

Llewellyn Publications is a registered trademark of Llewellyn Worldwide Ltd.

Library of Congress Cataloging-in-Publication Data
Names: Erickson, Lisa, author.
Title: Chakra empowerment for women : self-guided techniques for healing
    trauma, owning your power & finding overall wellness / Lisa Erickson.
Description: First edition. | Woodbury, Minnesota : Llewellyn Publications,
    2019. | Includes bibliographical references and index. | Summary: "A
    how-to manual of chakra-based activation exercises/meditations for women
    with a focus on women's issues, including health"—Provided by
    publisher.
Identifiers: LCCN 2019035855 (print) | LCCN 2019035856 (ebook) | ISBN
    9780738761404 (paperback) | ISBN 9780738761527 (ebook)
Subjects: LCSH: Chakras. | Mental healing. | Spiritual healing. |
    Women—Mental health. | Women—Health and hygiene—Alternative
    treatment.
Classification: LCC BF1442.C53 E75 2019 (print) | LCC BF1442.C53 (ebook)
    | DDC 131—dc23
LC record available at https://lccn.loc.gov/2019035855
LC ebook record available at https://lccn.loc.gov/2019035856

Llewellyn Publications
A Division of Llewellyn Worldwide Ltd.
2143 Wooddale Drive
Woodbury, MN 55125-2989
www.llewellyn.com

Printed in the United States of America

Forthcoming Books by Lisa Erickson

The Art & Science of Meditation

For the women who have shared their stories with me:
may you be heard, honored, and healed

Contents

Disclaimer

The information in this book is not intended to be used to diagnose or treat any medical or emotional condition. To address medical or therapeutic issues, please consult a licensed professional.

The author and publisher are not responsible for any conditions that require a licensed professional. Readers are encouraged to consult a professional with any questions about the use or efficacy of the techniques or insights in this book.

All case studies and descriptions of persons have been changed or altered so as to be unrecognizable. Any likeness to actual persons, living or dead, is strictly coincidental.

Foreword

Decades ago, I was under the tutelage of a Belizean shaman. One afternoon, after he explained the curative properties of various jungle plants, he smiled and leaned toward me, ignoring my male companions.

"I'm only teaching the men," he whispered. "You are a woman. You are aware of what I am speaking."

I was puzzled and asked the shaman, a natural herbal healer, what he meant.

"Women already know all things. Men must learn all things." He paused and pointed toward my abdomen. "There, that is why. You have the power of the Mother—and of all mothers."

Since that day, my awareness of the inner magic afforded the feminine has been increasingly heightened. Miraculously, Lisa's book speaks to this reality, the tradition of the feminine as anchored in mystery, mastery, and marvels. Rather than locating our personal power in the first chakra, the subtle energy center devoted to primal activity, we are rooted in the second chakra, the home of emotions, creativity, sensuality, and endless wisdom.

Lisa shares that all women, no matter how they identify in terms of sexuality, are like the lotus, a flower epitomizing the second chakra. The lotus is the sacred flower of India. The petals bloom upon long stalks that rise out of muddy waters. Representing purity, the lotus is able to detach from the murky desires that pull us down and enable service to higher forms of love. Each blossom opens to the streams of the sun, the moon, and the stars, receiving droplets of heaven with which we can remake the earth. My Belizean teacher of long ago had known this. His tribe understood that because women inhabit the second chakra, the womb-space, we hold a mini universe within us. Through each woman flows the knowledge of the Milky Way.

The problem is—and this is a huge problem—this knowledge isn't widely taught, even in energy medicine circles. Nearly every presentation of the energetic anatomy, the complex rendering of chakras, channels, and fields that compose our subtle body, accentuates the first chakra, the male center of power, as the fundamental chakra. Until Lisa's book, the positioning of the female power base has been largely ignored. This means that the solace, healing, and restitution that is promised through chakra-based systems has been unavailable to the very people who need it the most: women.

It is not biased or sexist to insist upon the need for a feminine-oriented energy system and set of applications. It is a necessity. Society has stripped women of their originality, self-esteem, and safety. It is women who bring future women and men into this world, and whose ability to spin peace out of cruelty is now required to save the very world that has demeaned them. It matters not if a woman has given birth to a third-dimensional child; the power of the womb gives all women the gift of creation.

Long overdue are the sacred understandings and exercises featured in Lisa's book. After all, for thousands of years, women have been disempowered and disenfranchised. During much of that time, women were considered the property of men, to be used as seen fit. Little wonder that the templates for the energetic systems forget the women. It is equally disturbing that in many places, women are still considered economic and political commodities, their powers repressed, their achievements unrecognized. Unfortunately, when the god in the mirror has a male face, to protest rape, violation, or harassment is to try and move forward against a headwind. These factors make it all the more important to repair and renew the subtle system.

In the last sentence, I used the word "repair" on purpose. As the words of the Belizean shaman suggest, our ancestors most likely perceived that the feminine and masculine are equivalent revelations of the Divine, emanations of a Creator that reflects both sets of qualities. Within a balanced presentation, all children are guaranteed care, no matter their gender or sexual preferences, for all genders are respectable. When the differences and similarities are recognized, the uniqueness of every individual can be cultivated. It is now time—past time—to resurrect what we know innately to be true, and we turn to Lisa's book to accomplish that feat.

I can testify to the distinctiveness of *Chakra Empowerment for Women* as I'm considered an expert on the subtle energy anatomy. I've written twenty-five books on related subjects and taught classes around the world. In fact, one of my books is twelve hundred pages long. The second half of that particular book features chakra systems from around the world. Nearly every system I've researched or studied has failed to address the differences between the female and male subtle anatomies. What was once written "by Spirit" has been written out.

There have been way-showers, to include authors like Diane Stein; I've even addressed the feminine variations on the energy system in a couple of my books. But besides depicting the importance of the feminine chakra system, Lisa's book also confronts the need for women to be healed from abuses of power. Moreover, it shows them how to do it. This is a book we want to collectively shout out about from every rooftop. This is a book every woman would benefit from reading—and employing.

To me, this truth is self-evident, not only because I understand energy, but because I was an English major. As such, I've read a lot of books. I was an undergraduate university student when I began to perceive that the feminine is truly different than the masculine, and that women's lives need to be defined and supported in ways unique to their gender. I became overtly aware of this truth during a semester devoted to women's literature.

Thirty women, sequestered together, took no other classes. We simply perused women's writings, many of the works resurrected from graves that had been dug by male professors, philosophers, and politicians. Some of the books were archaic, such as the works of Hildegard von Bingen, a German abbess who lived about a thousand years ago. How many people know that a woman was one of the founders of natural history, a woman who was simultaneously a philosopher, healer, herbalist, composer, mystic, and polymath? Other writings were more contemporary, including the passionate demands of Virginia Woolf, who decreed that the world would be improved if every woman could but have a "room of her own," a space for creative expression.

Eventually, our classroom became filled with symbols representing women's reality. The red cloths reminded us of the blood lost by the unlimited numbers of women who have been raped or killed as spoils of war and domestic violence. Earthen vases epitomized the original image of the Goddess, who was eventually dominated by warrior gods. Blues and purples embodied women's sacred knowledge and visions, which had been first maligned and then stolen by many of the religious. But the décor was secondary. The primary takeaway was that women's voices, so denounced, needed to be heard.

In *Chakra Empowerment for Women*, Lisa gives voice to what women have always known, and also what they must hear. She gives voice to the uniqueness of the feminine experience and the distinction of our subtle anatomy. She gives voice to our right to heal and the necessity for doing so.

It is time.

It is time for every woman everywhere to sing her own song; to bloom where she stands; to dance wildly; to create sublimely; to embrace joyfully; to cry stupendously; and to mother devotedly. And it is time for you to be aware of the universe within you and, through it, give birth to your own greatness.

Cyndi Dale

Introduction

The last few years have seen a surge of awareness and activity around women's empowerment in the social and political realm—the Women's Marches, #MeToo, and a record number of women running for elective office. Along with these external shifts has come a hunger for corresponding internal change and the tools to support this. This book is one such tool. It is a guide to the feminine energetic technology within you—a technology that you have always possessed to facilitate your own growth and healing. I believe learning to use it is your birthright.

With an increasing number of people turning to yoga, meditation, and other mind-body modalities for healing and wellness, the chakras have become more widely known. As energy centers that link mind, body, and spirit, the chakras provide multiple access points, and there are many corresponding methods for working with them. What's been given relatively little attention however, is how women might work with them differently from men. Just as our physical bodies differ, so do our energy bodies, and learning to work with these differences can be life-changing for women. I have designed the chakra tools in this book around these differences—what I have come to call Women's Energetics.

My own interest in Women's Energetics came with the birth of my first child. At that point I had already practiced chakra meditation daily for fifteen years and explored other aspects of the chakras through my energy healing training. But with the birth of my daughter, my energy body changed drastically, as did my relationship with my chakras. I went in search of new information to help me understand the shifts and how I could work with them. Buried in texts on tantra, "womb wisdom," and energy medicine treatments for women's health issues, I found variations in chakra placement and energy flow based on women's energy bodies. I began to experiment with chakra exercises based on these variations and develop my own set of tools.

Around the same time, I was seeing an increase in the number of women coming to me for help healing from sexual abuse and assault. Research indicates that one in five American girls are sexually abused before the age of seventeen, and one in six adult women are the victims of sexual assault. I found a much higher percentage of both in my own mostly female clientele. The correlation made sense to me because research has repeatedly shown a high correlation between sexual abuse, assault, and subsequent physical and mental health issues. While I am a firm believer in the power of talk therapy and other forms of counseling as well as medical treatment, I sought ways to complement these modalities for my clients with energy work, based on the principles of Women's Energetics I was exploring.

Over time I developed a free e-book, *Energy Work for Sexual Trauma,* which has been used by thousands of women. I developed a more targeted four-session teleseminar for healing sexual trauma that many hundreds of women have participated in over the last decade. I also developed a more general course on Women's Energetics for DailyOM, a website about holistic medicine and conscious living, and I continued my private session practice, and shared teachings on my blog, *Mommy Mystic.*

It is from all of this work, the thousands of women I have been privileged to work with, as well as my own personal experience, that this book has been born. I had five goals for myself as I wrote this book—five guiding principles:

- **Keep It Practical.** I want to help you *use* your chakras in daily life. This is a how-to, not a theoretical book. My goal is to provide relevant energy tools for you whether you are new to the chakras or have been working with them for years.
- **To the Point.** If there is one thing women are, it's *busy.* I have presented the 12 'Empowerments' in this book in a no-nonsense, consistent, easy to access fashion.
- **Specific to Women.** The tools you will learn in this book are adapted from Women's Energetics teachings, based on the feminine energy body and life phases.

- **Support Healing from Sexual Trauma.** Since so many women have experienced sexual trauma, and I believe all of us to some extent are impacted by the cultural baggage that has allowed it to flourish, I have emphasized ways to support this healing energetically.

- **Grounded in Love.** I wanted this book rooted in love. I love the chakras; I love the women I have been honored to work with; and I love the healing, empowerment, and awakening I have been privileged to witness in them.

This book is for you. I hope you find it healing, empowering, and awakening.

The Chakra Empowerments

In this book you will learn twelve chakra tools that I have called Empowerments because each is designed to bring forth a different power within you. You will learn how to bring forth these powers through an activation process involving visualization, spoken affirmations, and memory. While at first you will want to activate each Empowerment in a private, quiet space, with time you will be able to do so through on-the-spot shortcuts, in daily situations when you need to. In broad strokes, here are examples of how you might employ each Chakra Empowerment:

Root Bowl: to quell anxiety, develop stability, and increase vitality

Sacral Lotus: to spur creativity, problem solve, and heal the feminine

Navel Fire: to build confidence, determination, and focus

Heart Star: to improve connection with loved ones, find emotional balance, and lighten up

Throat Matrix: to communicate effectively, strengthen authenticity, and process feedback

Third Eye: to increase intuition, imagination, and insight

Crown Connection: to inspire faith, release self-doubt, and open spiritually

Second Skin: to affirm boundaries and protect yourself from energy loss

Web of Light: to improve relationships and release old dynamics

Feminine Pathway: to embrace change, and work with your feminine
cycles and phases

Healing Rays: to aid your own physical and emotional healing

Rainbow Abundance: to manifest your highest potential

In each case, once you have learned how to activate an Empowerment,
you can use it either in a moment of need to bring forth an energy quickly,
or as part of a daily routine for a period of time to facilitate lasting change.
For example, you might activate the Root Bowl to calm yourself down before
a job interview, the Navel Fire to charge yourself up before competing in a
sporting event, or the Heart Star before a difficult conversation with your
teenager. You may use Healing Rays to speed your recovery from a cold,
Second Skin to affirm boundaries before a large family gathering, or Web of
Light to let go of an old relationship. The possibilities are endless.

By activating a Chakra Empowerment, you can take control of the energy
and state of awareness you bring to a situation. In addition, if you feel that
you are chronically weak in an energy represented by a particular chakra or
are in a phase of life in which it is weakened, you can activate that Empowerment daily for a period of time to empower yourself. You might use the
Sacral Lotus every day for a month if you are a writer struggling with a block,
the Throat Matrix daily if you are working to improve communication with
your spouse, or Crown Connection regularly if you are feeling lost and seeking spiritual guidance. You might use Feminine Pathway together with Rainbow Abundance when you are working toward a big goal central to your
dreams for your life.

All of these Empowerments are customized based upon how a woman's
energy body works. In each chapter, I will outline for you key issues pertain-
ing to women and the chakras, along with ideas for how you might work with
an Empowerment to help you if these issues are relevant to you. I will also
outline how you can best use each Empowerment to support healing from
sexual abuse, assault, harassment or trauma. In later chapters I will talk about
how you can use some of the Empowerments in conjunction with menstruation, pregnancy, menopause, and other feminine cycles and transitions.

Chakra Basics

While this is a "doing" book rather than a theoretical one, you do need to know some basics about the chakras, and the chakra map I am using, in order to get started. Put simply, chakras are energy centers. They are intersections of energy currents within us. To access them, we focus on a physical location in our body, but it is not quite correct to say that they are "in" our physical body. The chakras are intersections between our mind, our body, and our spirit. You can define spirit however you like, but once you start connecting with the chakras, over time you will begin to experience this level of energy as palpably as you currently experience your five physical senses.

The word *chakra* is a Sanskrit word, usually translated as "wheel" or sometimes "wheel of light." Although the most well-known chakra mappings do originate from India, many other wisdom traditions around the world have or had energy center mappings. That most of these systems developed independently of each other (and many do not use the term "chakra"), and have numerous similarities is striking.

In this book I use the word "mapping" because I think it is most helpful to think of chakra systems as maps of the different kinds of energy that compose human life and consciousness. A map is not a place itself but a tool for navigating a place; the type of map you need varies according to your objectives. If you are visiting California, you might need a road map, a geological map, a hiking map, or a water access map. All of these maps are of California, but none of them are California itself. Each map provides a specific way for your mind to comprehend and navigate California based on what you are there to do.

The same is true of different energy body mappings, each one found around the world developed for a particular purpose. Some developed within meditation traditions and were designed to bring about enlightenment or mystic experience. Some developed within energy healing traditions in which the main focus was to bring energies into the physical body for the purposes of balance, regeneration, or speeding healing. Still other energy or chakra mappings developed as part of traditions that were trying to manipulate energies in the world—what we might consider to be magic. All of the mappings are valid, just like all the maps of California are valid, but we need to pick one to work with based on our purpose.

Though I work with several different energy body mappings in my own work, the Empowerments in this book are based on a well-known seven-chakra system that is familiar to those in the West. However, there are variations even in this system, particularly in the focal points for the lower three chakras. I have selected locations that best highlight the needs of women, and I'll explain why as we move through the chapters.

Following is an image of the main physical focal points for the chakra system we will use, along with some keywords representing the types of energies linked to each.

Chakra Access Points

Chakra	Focal Point	Energies
1 Root	Tailbone	Safety, stability, vitality
2 Sacral	Pelvis	Creativity, emotions, sensuality
3 Navel	Just under navel	Personal power, will, self
4 Heart	Center of upper chest	Compassion, balance, love
5 Throat	Center of neck	Expression, authenticity, clarity
6 Third Eye	Above brow midpoint	Insight, intuition, imagination
7 Crown	Top back part of head	Spirituality, faith, purpose

You will learn plenty about each chakra as you learn the Empowerments, so we will not go into much more detail; just know that there are many different ways to connect to and work with the chakras. In this book, we will work visually and with emotion through words—the latter in the form of affirmational statements to evoke emotions associated with each chakra. We will also work with your memory, as I will help you draw upon times in the past when you have already experienced the energies and state of awareness we are trying to bring forth with an Empowerment. If you are accustomed to working with the chakras already through other methods, such as yoga, pranayama breathing, Reiki healing, sound healing, crystals, or any other modality, you can easily combine these with the Chakra Empowerments activation steps. The Chakra Empowerments are based on visuals and affirmations to make

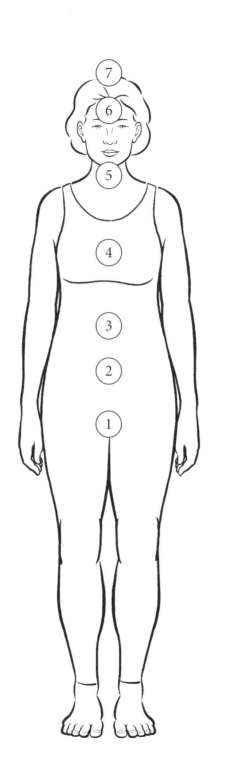

them easier to access in a moment on the go when you need to bring forward a particular energy right away. Initially, however, you will use them in a more meditative setting and can combine other chakra modalities at that time.

The main energetic differences between women's and men's energy bodies are in the first and second chakras, the ones whose focal points are in our lower body and pelvic area—of course also the location for the main physical differences between men and women. The primary difference is that men's energy bodies are anchored in their first chakras, and women's energy bodies are anchored in their second chakras. This difference affects energy flows throughout our entire subtle body, and the way we process energy coming into our subtle body from our environment and people around us. We will talk more about how these differences manifest throughout the book.

It is important to understand these energy body differences as part of a spectrum, not as absolutes. You may identify with some of what I say about women's energy bodies as true for you, and other aspects may not resonate. It is often unpopular today to talk about differences between men and women at all, because in the past they have been used to define women as the weaker sex and to discriminate accordingly. We also now understand gender as a social construct, as more people have come forward as transgender, gender-fluid, and gender neutral. The truth is that gender has always been a spectrum, not a fixed attribute.

Within the context of energetics, we need some framework for talking about the variety of patterns that exist in our energy bodies; because our energy body is an intermediary between our physical body and our psychological self, gender is a factor. I have personally found in my own client work that gender identity, as opposed to biological sex, is the most relevant factor in terms of how the chakras function. So if you identify as female, you will likely identify with much of what I say about Women's Energetics. If you identify as male, maybe not so much.

However, this is very individual, and I want you to honor your experience and intuition on the matter. I offer up these teachings on Women's Energetics to redress the imbalance that has occurred in most chakra teachings throughout the ages. For the most part, they have centered on men's experience of the chakras because the traditions that survived—or the teachings that survived in a form we can access—were male dominated.

One result of this predominance has been a lack of understanding of how specifically sexual abuse, assault, harassment, or any sort of sexually related trauma affects a woman's subtle body. We are at a moment in history in which there is finally a real push for change on a cultural level, and with that comes a growing opportunity for healing. Although there are many modalities available to help sexual trauma survivors, I have found that working with the chakras has much to offer. In each chapter I will offer ways to work with the Empowerment of that chapter within the context of sexual trauma healing. These Empowerments are meant to complement, not replace, other healing modalities such as therapy, support groups, body work, or medical and holistic health treatments.

Of course there are also many male victims of sexual abuse and assault. While the Empowerments in this book are designed for women based on our subtle bodies, for me the larger healing process is really about and for us all. If there is one thing that becomes very clear as you work with the chakras, it is that on the energetic level, we are all connected. When one of us engages in this work, it truly benefits us all. It creates a reverberation through the web of energy of which we are all a part. Women's empowerment can be men's liberation—from the cultural and historical restrictions placed on their own psyches and experience. So, my offering of these Empowerments is for our brothers, fathers, and sons, as much as for us, and our sisters, mothers, and daughters.

How to Use This Book

Each chapter begins with the Empowerment visual as you will imagine it in your own body. These visuals are available in full color in the book insert and are shown in the book on a generic female figure sitting cross-legged, but you may stand or sit in a chair if you prefer. Once you are familiar with activating an Empowerment, you may do so in more immediate circumstances—in a parked car, a bathroom stall, your desk at work, or even in a room full of people—through accessing what's called a snapshot memory. The full activation steps will help you develop this ability

Under the Empowerment image at the start of each chapter, you will find basic information about which chakra(s) the Empowerment uses, which energies it will bring forth within you, and what type of situations or emotions you might use this Empowerment to address in your day or life.

After the visual and Empowerment information, you will find the same sections in every chapter:

- *Overview:* A general introduction to this Empowerment, the chakra(s) it is based upon, the energies you are empowering when you activate it, and how you may want to use it.

- *When You Have Felt This Before:* Examples of situations and activities in which you may have experienced the energy of this Empowerment before. You can use these memories to help you in the activation process.

- *Activation Steps:* A step-by-step guide for activating the Empowerment. Guided audios of these steps for each Empowerment are also available for download as mp3 files on the book's website.

- *When You Are Blocked:* Examples of how blocks to this chakra or chakras may reflect in your life.

- *Using This Empowerment:* Examples of daily situations in which you might want to activate this Empowerment, and phases of your life in which you may want to activate it regularly to bring about shifts.

- *Women's Energetics:* The ways this Empowerment works with a woman's energy body as well as relevant principles of Women's Energetics. This section also covers blocks of the chakras associated with this Empowerment that women are particularly prone to experiencing.

- *Sexual Trauma Healing:* The ways that the chakras associated with this Empowerment may be blocked or wounded because of sexual abuse, assault, or trauma, and how you might use this Empowerment to aid you in your healing process if this is relevant for you. I encourage you to read this section even if you do not feel you have ever experienced sexual trauma, if for no other reason than the cultural conditioning we all have experienced and the ways working with the Empowerments may help you release this conditioning.

In addition to these sections within each Empowerment chapter, you will also find stories of two women presented as case studies to help you understand how you might benefit from using the Empowerment. These stories are abstracted from the lives of real women with whom I have worked, with all identifying details modified and multiple stories combined in some cases for greater clarity. I have included women in many different phases of their lives, including those impacted by sexual trauma.

It's very important that you honor your sense of what is right for you as you work with each Empowerment, especially if you have experienced trauma of any form in your life. I have designed these Empowerments to be trauma-sensitive, and you should feel free to adapt them further if you need to. If you find any part of the activation process uncomfortable or triggering for you, such as closing your eyes or saying the affirmations out loud, then modify according to what works for you. There is a certain amount of challenge with visualizing for everyone, so give it some time and understand that you do not need a perfect visualization to connect with the Empowerments. More than anything, the Empowerments are about *feeling*—the visualization, affirmations, and memories are all aids to cultivating this. We will each resonate with a different aspect of the activation process.

You may also feel free to relate to the chakras from within whatever spiritual or psychological framework works for you. Some individuals do not connect with the chakras as energy, but instead as archetypes for aspects of our psyche. You can relate to the Empowerments in this way, and they will be just as effective for you. In terms of religion, I consider the chakras to be beyond any particular tradition, like a technology available to us all; therefore, I try not to project any particular religious or spiritual framework on the Empowerments in this book. You may add that, of course, and at certain points I will suggest how to do so.

It is most helpful to learn the Empowerments in order and work with each one for a period of time before moving on. The first seven Empowerments focus on one chakra each and provide a foundation for the later Empowerments. I suggest learning and utilizing one Empowerment a week over the course of twelve weeks. However, if you read through the entire book and feel that there are one or two Empowerments you really want to focus on, that is fine too. They are each designed to be activated independently.

Of course, it is important to remember that none of these Empowerments is a substitute for medical care, for mental health counseling, or for a qualified spiritual guide. These Empowerments are meant to be complements to all of those resources. Especially if you are working with these Empowerments as an aid to sexual trauma healing, please make sure you have all the support you need. At the same time, this is about self-empowerment, and you have more resources within you than you are likely aware of. Activating the Chakra Empowerments is part of what will help you to connect with these inner resources.

Final Advice

Dive in! This book is about direct experience, an immersion approach to learning to work with your chakras. In this introduction I have offered you information that may be helpful but do realize that the key to all of these Empowerments is already in you. You have a deep knowing about how to use them. All I am trying to offer you are the triggers and guidance you need to bring that healing forth. Experiment and trust yourself.

ONE
Root Bowl: Your Foundation

Related Chakras: Your root, or first, chakra

Energies: Grounding, safety, security, support, presence, vitality, stability, resilience

Use For: Anxiety, instability, overwhelm, spacey-ness, disassociation, feeling unsupported, fatigue

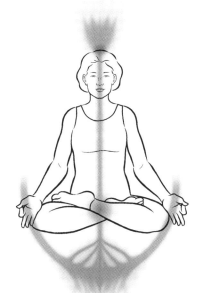

Like the foundation of a house, your root chakra is your energetic foundation. Its most important function is to support your ability to feel safe in your body. When we don't feel safe, everything is defined by our fear and we can do little but react. We ordinarily think of this in terms of physical danger—if we are about to be attacked by a tiger, our body and our psyche will react in one of three ways—fight, flight, or freeze. But we have these reactions in our daily lives, even when there is no mortal threat. They can as a result limit our ability to respond effectively and productively to a situation.

For example, say a coworker criticizes something you do in front of your supervisor, and you feel as if she is trying to undermine you. You feel threatened, triggering feelings of anxiety. When you next see this coworker, these feelings rise up and you may become angry and combative (fight), tongue-tied and unable to respond (freeze), or seek to escape the encounter as quickly as possible (flight). None of these reactions helps you to respond in the most effective manner—to deal with your coworker maturely and strategically.

Feeling safe is the foundation for our ability to respond effectively to any situation. Feeling safe enables *choice*. It allows us to respond from a place of self-awareness so that we can choose our response. Believing in our ability to choose an effective response in turn serves as the basis for resilience, our faith in ourselves to handle anything that arises. When we believe in our own resilience, we are able to meet the world fearlessly. We trust ourselves to handle whatever comes our way.

This self-trust, this belief in our resilience, not only provides a strong foundation for our psyche and mental health but also for our body and physical health. We now know that chronic stress and anxiety take an immense toll. Our body reacts to stress by raising levels of certain hormones that aid our body's ability to react quickly and strongly in cases of real danger, but persistent high levels of these hormones are linked to many health problems. Our ability to respond to difficult situations in our lives calmly, rooted in self-trust and faith in our resilience, can help prevent our body triggering the stress response linked to these conditions. If you have experienced trauma in your life, you may have particular difficulty tapping into these feelings of safety, self-trust, and resilience, increasing your risk for stress-based issues.

The purpose of the Root Bowl Empowerment is to help you connect with these feelings in any moment; if you choose to work with it longer term, it will help you strengthen your overall energetic and psychological foundation. When this foundation is strong, other energies associated with our root become more available to us, including its role in our ability to manifest goals. Our root chakra is linked to our ability to bring things into being, to make things happen in our life. We start with an idea, with something in our head, and in order to make it real and present, we have to bring it down into reality—we have to *ground* it. The energies of our first chakra are what allow us to give something roots in this way.

The Root Bowl is an essential foundational Empowerment: it will help you generate the energy of safety necessary to empower your sense of resilience and choice, allow your body to stay calm and healthy when challenges arise, and fuel your ability to make your dreams and goals a manifest reality.

Lauren was twenty-seven and very spiritually inclined, but had cycled through a series of dead-end jobs and was never been able to attain any financial security. She had no trouble getting hired, and each job would start out OK, but eventually some personal conflict would arise with a coworker or her boss and her performance would start to suffer. She would begin to arrive late or leave early, her attitude and work relationships soured, and eventually she would be let go or leave before she could be.

In working with Lauren, we focused on her feelings when conflict arose with coworkers. Even a small unpleasant encounter would trigger anxiety for her, and she would spin for hours about what she should have said or how unjust the situation was. Though she also avoided conflict in her personal life, it was particularly pronounced at work.

She began doing the Root Bowl for ten minutes every day, focusing on cultivating feelings of safety and resilience. Then she began working with the Root Bowl for a couple of minutes in the bathroom after any incident at work that triggered feelings of anxiety or anger. Eventually, she began flashing on the Root Bowl within incidents in which she found herself feeling anxious or defensive. She worked to cultivate her ability to stay calm and choose her response. In situations that did not go well, she would activate the Root Bowl and return to the person to try to hash things out after the fact.

Lauren began to trust in her ability to withstand negativity and to counter or shift interactions. She also began therapy to explore how these patterns had developed. As Lauren's sense of her own resilience and self-understanding grew, she was able to relax in confrontational situations and let them go after they arose or deal with them effectively. For the first time she was able to hold a job long enough to get promoted and see a path to financial stability.

Many women have difficulty with confrontation or negativity, due to prevalent "nice girl" conditioning. If you have any history of abuse in your background, this may be magnified, as you seek safety by placating those around you. If you are energetically sensitive, you may also have difficulty letting go of the negative energies and emotions generated in such encounters. Perhaps you go straight to anger as a protective measure, simply remove yourself from the situation, or swing between the two as in Lauren's case.

Working with the Root Bowl can be a powerful way of developing the energies of safety, security, resilience, and self-trust that you need to shift this pattern. Other Empowerments in this book, such as Second Skin and Navel Fire, may be of help too. We will cover how some of these Empowerments work together as we move through this book.

When You Have Felt This Before

A key part of activating each Chakra Empowerment is learning to use the power of memory to remember times in which you have already felt the corresponding states before. After all, your chakras have been active every moment of your life; they haven't just been waiting for you to notice them! You can use the power of your memories to tune into feelings you've had in the past and use them to activate an Empowerment more quickly.

For example, do you have a person in whose presence you feel absolutely safe and trusting? A person with whom you don't feel as if you have to pretend to be anyone other than who you are? With this person, you feel as if you can just be yourself and that no matter what, this person will have your back. If you have someone like this in your life, it serves as a good example of the kind of relaxation, ease, and sense of security that is generated by the Root Bowl; you can also draw upon memories of being with this person during the activation process.

Another possibility relevant to the Root Bowl is any memories you have of feeling particularly strong and present in your body. If you are an athlete, avid exerciser, or dancer (even dancing around in your living room by yourself counts, which I highly recommend) and during these activities feel profoundly present in your body or "in the zone," this is also something you may draw upon. These are moments of absolute trust in your body, moments of spontaneously experiencing physicality that feels *safe*. In these moments, your body is free of anxiety.

This relationship with physicality and feeling of absolute presence also often arises in nature. One common way of working with the chakras is through the elements, and the root chakra is linked to the element of earth. Spending time walking in nature, particularly in environments with rich soil and lots of healthy trees or other plant life, is especially likely to generate powerful root chakra energies. Because of the link to the body and exercise, rigorous outdoor earth-based activities such as mountain climbing and canyoneering are also very likely to connect you with these energies. They combine physical one-pointed focus with connecting to the element of earth, together activating the feelings associated with your root chakra.

Closely related to the root chakra's connection to earth is the concept of *grounding*. Grounding in our energy bodies is very similar to grounding an electrical current—it means that our energy is plugged into, and anchored by, a stabilizing force. When we are grounded, we feel fully present in and attuned to our body—our mind is not spinning off uncontrollably. We are not thinking about the past or the future. We are right in the present moment with everything it has to offer, no matter if we consider the particular moment wonderful or terrible. If you can relate to times in your life in which you have felt very grounded and present in this way, then this is a powerful memory to draw upon when working to activate the Root Bowl.

It is perfectly OK if you cannot think of any examples such as these. Memories are a useful aid, but none of them fully express the power of the Root Bowl when it is fully activated. If you are able to surface one or two memories like these examples, you may want to jot them down for use when you are working with the activation steps in the next section. If you cannot think of any, then that may be a sign that you could benefit from working with the Root Bowl more regularly for a period of time, something we will talk about in a later section.

Activation Steps

Since this is our first activation process, here are a few tips on how best to prepare yourself (these will apply to all the Empowerments):

- Sit in a quiet, private space.

- Sit with your spine as erect as you are able to, in either a chair or on a cushion on the floor. Using cushions behind your back to support you is perfectly fine.

- If you are using memories from the When You Have Felt This Before section, remind yourself of what these are; you may have them jotted down next to you if you like.

- If you are using the guided audio file from the book website to guide you, get that queued up to play.

- Gaze at the image of the Root Bowl in the book insert until you feel familiar with it, and read through these instructions in entirety once before you begin.

- Most people find closing their eyes at each step is the most effective way to visualize, but if you feel uncomfortable in any way with your eyes closed, feel free to keep them slightly open, allowing your gaze to rest on a spot on the floor in front of you without focusing. Visualizing happens in your mind's eye, so this will not prevent you from doing so.

- Remember to be patient and nonjudgmental with yourself. It may take some time for you to really feel or imagine the Root Bowl to feel as if it is activating. With practice, you will get better and faster, and eventually will need just a second of visualizing or stating an affirmation to feel it is fully activated.

- Honor your feelings. If you feel triggered, anxious, or uncomfortable, take a break, modify the process, or try again another day. Feel free to adapt this activation process, and draw upon the aspects of it that are the most effective for you. This is your process, so trust your own intuition about what is right for you.

Once you have prepared yourself in these ways, you can begin the activation steps.

Step 1: Imagine a beautiful red light deep below you in the earth, beneath the foundation of whatever building you are in, however far down that may be, even if you are in a high-rise. Go all the way down into the earth and imagine a brilliant, vibrant red light.

Step 2: See this vibrant red light emanating upward through the earth as a column of red light, gently radiating up into your tailbone at the very base of your spine. You may place your hand on your tailbone and imagine a ball of red light growing brighter there as you do so.

Step 3: Then imagine, back down in the earth just beneath you, some of the red light is branching off from the column rising up from the depths of the earth and forming a bowl all around you. Imagine you are sitting in a beautiful bowl made of radiant red light. This bowl feels like it is supporting and protecting you on all sides.

Step. 4: When you feel ready to move on, imagine the light from your tailbone is now moving all the way up through your body, up the center of your torso, enlivening and energizing you as it does so. It's moving up through your belly, your chest, your neck, your throat, the top of your head.

Step 5: See this entire visual and hold it: a red light comes up from the earth; part of it comes up into your tailbone and from there rises all the way up through the center of your body to the crown of your head. Part of the light emanates out around you and creates a bowl in which you are sitting. In this bowl you feel safe, secure, protected, and held.

Step 6: If you are working with memories, bring them to mind now. Cycle through each one, holding them in your mind until the associated feelings arise within you. Then return your focus to the visual.

Step 7: Say each of the affirmations associated with this Empowerment one to three times, striving to feel what you are saying as you do so:

> I am safe.
> I am supported.
> I am energized.
> I am grounded.
> I am resilient.
> I love my body.

Step 8: Affirm the visual one more time and note how you are feeling. Imagine you are taking a snapshot in your mind of yourself with the Root Bowl fully activated—beginning to create the shortcut to activating this feeling more quickly in the future. This is your snapshot memory.

As with all the Empowerments, the activation occurs through the combination of building the visual step by step and generating associated feelings through the memories and affirmations. Really try to cultivate this sense that the earth is rising up to hold you, that it is creating this bowl in which you are sitting, and in which you are protected, supported, safe, and secure. Also connect with the enlivening, vibrant life energy coming up from the earth into your tailbone and energizing your entire body, like through the roots of a tree. This energy comes up into your energy body just like nutrients and water come up from the soil through the roots of a tree.

Of course at first this may all seem like a lot of work, and it may be hard to imagine you could ever activate an Empowerment in the moment you need it during your day. But with time you will create your own shortcut—that snapshot you take in the final step will translate into your ability to shift, and bring these energies forth, with a simple moment of visualization or affirmation whenever you need to do so.

When You Are Blocked

One of the main ways a blocked or weak root chakra may manifest in you is feeling spacey or disconnected from what is going on around you. An empowered root chakra creates a feeling of full presence; when it is weak, we feel the opposite. You may feel like you cannot focus, like your mind is jumping randomly from one thought to another. Or you may feel spaced out or checked out, perhaps losing blocks of time staring into space, or escaping the present mentally through incessant daydreaming. More severe forms of escapism could include excessive television watching, video gaming, or in the most damaging cases, substance abuse.

There is a spectrum of ways that we may disconnect, but all of them have to do with not being present in our body, and seeking to escape the present moment. Of course we all need diversions at times, and there is a role for fun escapism in our lives. It is only when these diversions are chronic, rising to the level of addiction or preventing us from accomplishing goals or actively participating in our lives, that it is a sign of a blocked or weak root chakra.

The other main way that a root chakra block or weakness may manifest is as constant anxiety. Anxiety relates to several chakras (and we will talk about it again in other chapters), but in the root chakra in particular, it may express as a chronic anxiety in which we never feel safe or relaxed. In particular, it may manifest as physical anxiety, impacting your health and your ability to connect with your physical body through exercise and self-care.

A third potential sign of problems with your root chakra is if you have chronic difficulty making things happen in your life, especially in relation to material areas like work, money, and a secure home. Of course, issues like these (e.g., health or money) are complicated and cannot be reduced to a single block in your energy body. Working through them may require working on several fronts. Certainly, working with the Root Bowl will help and can be part of the solution.

All of us may experience spacey-ness, anxiety, or difficulty achieving material goals at times, and this does not mean we have a weak or blocked root chakra. In situations where you are experiencing any of these, working with the Root Bowl in the moment will help you to break through and shift into a more productive and energized place. However, if you do feel as if any or all of these are a chronic problem for you, you may want to consider working with the Root Bowl as part of a more long-term personal development process. The next section gives ideas for how you might work with the Root Bowl in either capacity.

Using the Root Bowl

One way to think about using a Chakra Empowerment in your day is medicinal: What energy do you need or awareness field do you want to shift into to address a problematic or inhibiting feeling you are having in the moment? When you have a headache, perhaps you take aspirin; when you have heartburn, perhaps an antacid. Or maybe you prefer holistic approaches and you diffuse lavender essential oil or drink some peppermint tea. You can use Chakra Empowerments within your day in much the same way—to bring forth an energy or awareness counter to one that is causing you discomfort.

By now you understand the kinds of energies that the Root Bowl is meant to bring forth and address. Considering these, here are some examples of situations in which you may want to activate it on the spot in your day:

- Per our example in the first section, you hear that a coworker has said something critical of your work to your supervisor, and you feel threatened, anxious, or angry. Take a few minutes to activate the Root Bowl, and then think about the situation again, strategizing about how you can best respond. Activate the Root Bowl again right before the next time you know you will see this person.

- You are about to call a client, relative, or even friend that you know often upsets you or stresses you. Activate the Root Bowl before your call.

- Activate the Root Bowl anytime you are experiencing anticipatory nerves—before a big presentation, job interview, performance, medical procedure, difficult conversation, or other anxiety-producing event.

- After a stressful drive in traffic, a near accident, an argument, or a confrontation, use the Root Bowl to reestablish a sense of safety and transition into the next event of your day.

- If you feel overwhelmed, frenetic, or unfocused, activate the Root Bowl to ground yourself.

- If you find yourself spacing out, or craving escape at a time in which you need to focus, use the Root Bowl to reestablish a connection to the present.

As you get more comfortable with the Empowerments, you may find you wish to combine them, activating one first and then another. For example, if you are heading into a big presentation or job interview, you may want to activate the Root Bowl to calm yourself down, followed by the Navel Fire to bring forth your personal power and focus. Or if you are facing a difficult conversation with your rebellious teenage son, you may want to use the Root Bowl to soothe your nerves, followed by the Heart Star to center yourself in your maternal love and compassion for him. Keep it simple at first, but over time trust your intuition about how best to combine Empowerments to bring forth what you need within yourself.

If you feel that root chakra functions have been difficult for you to access throughout your life, you can work with the Root Bowl regularly for a period of time to help you to heal and unblock these energies. My recommendation is to activate an Empowerment for at least ten minutes a day for thirty days whenever you would like to focus in this way. However, you can adapt this to establish a goal that is realistic for you, maybe three times a week for five minutes over two months instead. If you are working your way through this book one Empowerment per week, I recommend completing that first, and then deciding which, if any, Empowerments you would like to spend a longer time with.

When you are working with an Empowerment longer term, often insights will arise related to why this chakra's energy is difficult for you to access. You may want to combine this work with journaling, counseling, life coaching, or healing modalities that support efforts to shift the habits and tendencies you are working on. But chakra work also has its own power and shifts often occur without mental analysis or processing. That is not to say that the work does not benefit from analysis, as it certainly does, and I find chakra work and talk-based therapy a particularly powerful combination. But for many people the Empowerments in this book are a gentle yet effective way of increasing energies in your awareness on their own.

You may have read about clearing, balancing, or opening your chakras. These are all different ways of working with your energy body; some are more focused on the connection between the chakras and the physical body, while others center on the psychological or spiritual aspects. It's important to understand that any clearing, balancing, or opening is not necessarily on every level, nor is it permanent. Often such work is like taking a bath—your chakras may be cleaned on the physical-auric level, or opened on the psychological or spiritual level for a period of time, but if you are thrust into a situation in which underlying obstructive patterns are triggered—in the case of the root chakra, if extreme anxiety, escapism, fatigue, or illness arise—the chakra may constrict or a new block may rise up. This is where the Chakra Empowerments become valuable, as they are meant to empower you to work with your chakras on your own when you need to throughout your life.

Here are some examples of when and why you may want to work with the Root Bowl regularly for an extended period:

- If you are going through a rehab or other substance abuse treatment program, working with the Root Bowl will provide you additional grounding and stabilizing support.

- If you feel you escape too much into television, gaming, the internet, or any other means of media and would like to increase your ability to stay present in your body in the moment.

- If you are struggling with constant anxiety or going through a particularly anxious period in your life. Of course, the Root Bowl cannot replace qualified mental health counseling or needed medication, but it may complement these means if they are required.

- If you are undergoing medical treatment for an illness or feel chronically fatigued.

- If you are embarking upon a new exercise regiment or weight loss program, the Root Bowl can help to empower your relationship with your physical body.

Again, these are just some examples, and as with the daily use examples, you may choose to combine your longer term work with work on other Empowerments at the same time. More examples are provided in subsequent chapters.

Women's Energetics: Body Connection

Men's energy bodies are anchored in their root chakra, while ours are anchored in our second, or sacral, chakra. One of the by-products is that the energies and psychological aspects of the root chakra are usually more central to a man's coming into his personal power and identity in the world, while for women the energies and themes of our sacral are more central. Our power on the subtle body level is entwined with the energies of our sacral chakra; working on empowering this chakra will do more for us than any other. For this reason, we will delve more deeply into the main principles of Women's Energetics and the feminine subtle body in the next chapter.

However, our subtle body is a balanced system, and the chakras are meant to be worked with holistically. The health and empowerment of each is necessary for our health and empowerment as a whole, so it is critical that women work on strengthening our root chakras, even more so because historically and culturally we have all too often been prevented from fully owning the powers of this chakra as our own.

To some extent, the root chakra represents the physical, and the second chakra represents the emotional. Historically men have been granted the physical as their arena, and women the emotional as ours. It has been reflected in power structures originally founded on the physical dominance of men, perpetuated long term through cultural and institutionalized sexism, and it has been damaging to all of us. Emotional balance and well-being, as well as women's sexual and procreative energies have been denigrated and even demonized. Men have been cut off from the healthy expression of their sacral energies, and women from the healthy empowerment of their root chakra energies.

At this time in history, these patterns are thankfully (though at times painfully) changing, and we are all a part of it. For women today, focusing on healing and empowering our root chakra is especially important, and it is supported by the larger energetic shifts occurring. I find that the most important aspect of this work has to do with healing our relationship with our body. We receive a lot of negative messages related to our body: that we are not as strong as boys or men and that it's a problem; that one aspect of being in a woman's body—menstruation—is at best a nuisance and at worst a curse; and, most problematically, that a lot of our worth rests on how our body *looks*. Although both men and women are held to standards regarding physical appearance, for women it is especially pronounced.

In short, we are often conditioned to believe that our body is a problem. It is either not strong enough, thin enough, or pretty enough, or it is inconveniencing us, holding us back. We are left feeling our body is a problem we need to solve or something we need to change. This undercurrent creates a rift in our root chakra energies—our root chakra is about full presence in the moment, and that includes feeling fully present in our bodies. If we are not comfortable with our bodies, we are often incapable of being fully present in them or of fully inhabiting them.

A big part of root chakra work for women, therefore, is focusing on generating *body love*. Surface and release the judgements you have about your body, especially regarding body image, and focus on all your body does for you instead. Make a list of the aspects of your body that are strong, or that are your favorites, from an exercise, health, and beauty perspective. Perhaps you have always had strong legs but spend a lot of time judging how thick they are. Focus on their strength and express gratitude for it. Perhaps you rarely get sick—focus on gratitude for your strong immune system. Think too of all the activities you enjoy in your body—perhaps you like to hike or engage in other outdoor activities. Even enjoying a warm bath or massage counts—after all, how would you experience that without your body? There are countless pleasures and experiences our body enables us to have. Shifting into a relationship of gratitude for these can help us to shift our relationship with our body.

Gratitude and body love do not mean you should avoid focusing on body related changes, especially those related to your health, such as increased exercise, improved diet, or even weight loss if it is needed. The goal instead is to shift your intention and motivation as you do so. Engage in these as acts of body love rather than body-hate. They are acts of self-care rather than self-judgment. Even beauty appointments and changes can be approached in this way, as acts of bringing forth and celebrating your true beauty, as opposed to covering or altering that which is "ugly."

Shifting this relationship with your body will help to empower all of the other aspects of your root chakra and support your ability to fully activate the Root Bowl. Fully inhabiting your body will increase your ability to bring forth the Root Bowl's energies of calm, grounding, security, stability, and vitality. This in turn will empower the sense of self-trust, resilience, and freedom to choose your responses in situations. For women, changing our relationship to our body is key to generating the empowered energetic foundation we need to thrive and grow. That foundation will form the base for any of the other energetic work you choose to engage in through the Empowerments.

Marie was thirty-six and had just gone through a difficult breakup. She was a successful marketing executive who wanted marriage and children, but she had never had a relationship that lasted for longer than a year. She had grown up in a home with an alcoholic father and was sexually abused by an uncle who came to live with them for several months when she was eight years old. She had worked with a therapist for several years in her late twenties as well as Al-Anon to help her work through the related emotional scars. Although this work had helped her greatly, she felt she had a wall up in personal relationships that she could not surmount.

Marie wanted to focus on opening her heart chakra, as she felt she was not able to open and connect in relationships. I encouraged her to work with the Root Bowl for a period of time, first laying the foundation of safety and self-trust necessary to begin to open to others. At first, Marie found it very difficult to feel the energy of safety, security, and resilience. She realized that these feelings were entirely foreign to her, and that in fact, she walked around all the time on guard, looking for potential threats. Although she could connect with feeling grounded, the feelings of safety and resilience and the resultant self-trust and relaxation were very new for her.

Marie also found herself resistant to body love affirmations. Healthy and fit, she had not perceived herself as having a poor body image, but in fact was highly critical of her perceived physical "flaws" and mostly related to her body and its cycles as things she had to put up with. After working on connecting to these cycles, body love, and the Root Bowl for several weeks, Marie first noticed she was more humorous and spontaneous with her coworkers. She was beginning to relax, and it was thus reflected in her social interactions. She also inhabited her body in a new way, such that a friend noticed and complimented her on it.

With time, we did work on other chakras together, including Marie's heart. Her next relationship was with a very different kind of man, and she was very different in the relationship. She realized that because in the past she had not truly felt safe enough to open to a deep heart connection, she had been attracted to men who she intuitively knew were also not capable of this. As she shifted, so did the type of people she felt drawn to. As of this writing, Marie and her new beau are going strong and very much in love.

Women often feel they need to work on their heart chakras after a relationship has gone bad or if they are having a hard time meeting potential partners. We are often conditioned to take responsibility for everything that happens in a relationship; even after leaving an abusive relationship, we will sometimes blame ourselves or believe we were at fault for "attracting" an abusive partner or were not nurturing enough to heal our partner's damage. Like Marie, many women feel that they need to be more open, loving, and pure in their hearts in order to attract the right partner.

In fact, more often there are patterns of anxiety and self-worth that need to be addressed—root and sacral chakra issues—more than those of the heart. The lower chakras are the foundation for our energy body; psychologically, they represent the solid ground upon which a healthy psyche is formed. It is often after working to cultivate the energies of one or both of these chakras that we will generate shifts throughout our entire subtle body and psyche, as in Marie's case.

Sexual Trauma Healing: Feeling Safe and Staying Present

Healing your relationship with your body is even more central to working with the Root Bowl if you have experienced sexual abuse, assault, harassment, or any form of sexual trauma. Perhaps your abuser or assaulter made you feel as if you or your body were to blame for the abuse or assault. Perhaps you received victim-blaming messages from individuals you confided in or from the media at large. Perhaps you simply cannot relate to your body because you view it as the site of your trauma or feel as though it betrayed you.

These feelings play out for victims—or survivors, the term I prefer—in a number of ways. Some women experience health issues stemming from lack of self-care or self-abuse. Others are driven to hide their body through layers, baggy clothing, or weight gain. Some may develop eating disorders leading to unhealthy weight loss in an effort to disappear from view. Still others experience such acute body self-consciousness that they embark on endless regimes to improve their appearance and body shape but never feel satisfied with the result. Whatever the pattern, the heart of the issue is a disconnection or even hatred of their own body that also hinders the ability to connect with root chakra energies and their associated aspects—the sense of safety, security, grounding, vitality, and resilience.

So although focusing on body acceptance and body love is important for all women, it is especially important for you if you are a sexual trauma survivor. This may include identifying feelings of shame or self-blame that you have internalized. From an energetic perspective, these feelings are more related to the second chakra and will be discussed more in the next chapter, but it is important here to acknowledge when you need help facing and letting go of these feelings.

Another way the root chakra is affected by sexual trauma is the difficulty in accessing feelings of safety and security. Often when I am working with a survivor on the Root Bowl or related Empowerments, at some point she will say, "But what if I am actually *not* safe?" The reality is that if you have experienced sexual abuse or assault, you already know that your safety is not guaranteed all the time. If you experienced abuse as a child, you may have never developed a strong feeling of being safe and secure in the world; perhaps one of the adults tasked with keeping you safe was actually your abuser (as is common). If your assault occurred later, then any sense of safety and security may have been destroyed.

Any traumatic experience can have this effect, but for sexual trauma survivors it is often very pronounced because the vast majority of sexual assaults are perpetrated by individuals we know. These predators undermine not only our sense of safety in the world at large but also our sense of trust in those around us and our ability to judge people. As we have already explored, self-trust and a sense of safety are linked, together forming the foundation for our sense of our own resilience. As a result, sexual trauma undermines your ability to access this entire spectrum of root chakra energies.

With the Root Bowl, you are bringing forth the feeling of safety and security to access when you actually *are* safe. The result of trauma is often that we feel unsafe all the time and react from a place of "fight, flight, or freeze" when there is no actual threat. Living in this heightened state of anxiety and vigilance limits your ability to deal with everyday situations effectively and damages your health and stability. The Root Bowl is one Empowerment for helping you to begin to break this cycle.

Feeling unsafe may also be linked to spacey-ness or escapist tendencies such as those we have already talked about in relation to a blocked or weak root chakra. For sexual trauma survivors, it may present as more serious patterns of disassociation. During an assault or abusive episode, a victim's self-protective instincts may manifest as efforts to disassociate in the form of blacking out, moving in their minds to an untouchable place, or engaging in mental activity such as repetitive recitation of words or songs in order to disassociate from the traumatic bodily experience of the present. This can become a pattern that continues after the abuse or assault has ended. Disassociation can be escapism into drugs, alcohol, TV, video games, and so on, or it can reflect in a more subtle way, perhaps as a habit of always being in your mind, always worrying, or even always staying busy. Really, anything that takes you out of the present moment to a limiting degree can be a form of disassociation. Breaking deep-seated patterns of disassociation often requires professional help, but root chakra support through activating the Root Bowl is a powerful ally in that process.

One special note when working with the Root Bowl if you do feel you have patterns of disassociation: from an energetic perspective, disassociation is a tendency to live in the upper chakras without a balanced anchor in the lower chakras. There is a tendency to avoid focusing on the lower chakras and to feel more comfortable in the mental and upper energetic realms. Sometimes this tendency manifests as difficulty and discomfort when focusing on the lower chakras or even simply on the lower part of the body. If you experience this, please know that working through it is simply a natural part of the process of learning to activate this Empowerment. Begin lightly and gently with short periods of focus on the Root Bowl. Never push yourself—

stop if you feel overwhelmed or upset. You will likely find that with time, patience, and self-compassion your comfort level with this Empowerment will grow, and you will begin to experience the associated energy.

If you do not find it is getting easier, that is okay—*there is nothing wrong with you.* It is very important to remember this, as trauma survivors often internalize the idea that they have been irreparably damaged and nothing will work to help them. Perhaps what you need is more support, to proceed more slowly, or to adapt the activation steps. Or perhaps another Empowerment will work better for you—different Empowerments work for different individuals, or even different modalities. I encourage you to continue seeking what works for you. I have offered additional resources that may help you on the book website.

TWO
Sacral Lotus:
Your Inspiration

Related Chakras: Your second, or sacral, chakra

Energies: Inspiration, creativity, passion, sensuality, fluidity, adaptability, sexuality, feminine power

Use For: Rigidity, depression, emotional numbness, disconnection, problem-solving, feeling stuck or blocked, to spur creativity, to connect with feminine power, to spark sexuality

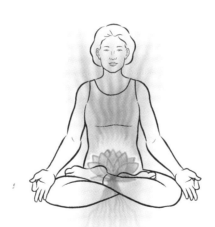

If you engage with only one Empowerment in this book, make it this one! The Sacral Lotus empowers your second, or sacral, chakra; it is the anchor for your feminine energy body. Likewise, the Sacral Lotus Empowerment affects your entire subtle body, not only your second chakra. Throughout history, many expressions of feminine second chakra energy have been denigrated and devalued. Learning to value and cultivate these energies is central to the healing shift our society needs as a whole right now within both men *and* women. And as a woman, bringing these forth within yourself is especially critical to your well-being.

Our sacral chakra energies provide the flow, connection, and inspiration in our life. This chakra provides life's juiciness—when these energies are flowing, we experience the world as vibrant, colorful, flavorful, and ripe … like the perfect piece of fruit. Whenever we feel excited or inspired by an idea, person, or something we have read, witnessed, or heard, the energies of this chakra have been activated. When we experience pleasure in any form, whether through a beautiful sunset, a delicious dessert, or a gentle touch, sacral chakra energies are strong. When we feel connected to others emotionally or physically, in sync with them on any level, this is also linked to sacral energies.

Because this chakra is linked to the internal reproductive organs and glands within most energy mapping systems, it is often thought of as either the sex chakra or the procreation chakra. Certainly, both birthing and sexual energy (especially feminine sexual energy) are linked to this chakra, which is part of the reason its energies have been historically devalued or even demonized within patriarchal cultures. However, a true understanding of this link requires expanding our view of both sexuality and birthing beyond the physical.

Let's take sexuality first—what is sexual desire as an energy? It is a drive to connect with the person we desire. It may be mixed up with other emotions, but at an energetic level, it is a striving for connection. In the moment of connection—when the desirer meets the desired—we feel temporarily satisfied, satiated, or even whole.

This movement toward connection is one of the primary energies of the sacral chakra, and sexual energy is just one expression of it. Really, this energy is what drives us to engage with the world—our desire to connect with people, sights, sounds, foods, places, experiences and more are all rooted in this sacral energy. While root chakra energy is static and represents stability and safety, sacral chakra energy represents our reaching outward from ourselves into the world. Sacral energy is the branches of a tree, reaching toward the sun and swaying in the breeze, while the roots stretch down into the earth and create a stable foundation. A healthy balance between the two is essential—a top-heavy tree with little root support will blow over in a storm, while a tree lacking branches will be unable to absorb the sunlight it needs to survive, nor will it blossom or bloom.

Blossoming and blooming culminate in birthing, the other primary energy of the sacral chakra. To truly understand it, we need to also look at birthing beyond the level of the physical. When we birth a child, we are bringing a being into the world that begins in our own body, as part of us. But through the act of birthing, it becomes separate, its own entity. This is what birthing is—the drive to create something separate from ourselves. All forms of creativity are birthing in this sense, whether we create a child, a painting, a book, an app, or a business. When we create, we are bringing something forth from ourselves and letting it go out into the world.

Connecting to and creating in the world are the essence of the second chakra, and from these the juiciness of life arises … as well as the spontaneity. This chakra isn't about rules and structure but about pleasure and passion in the moment, flow and pushing boundaries. It is about how something *feels* and is linked to our emotional life. It is also about cycles, the ebb and flow of energies in time, in our bodies, in our emotions. It is about movement and change. We need change, life is change, but it is in our nature to resist this. The fear of change and transience are part of what has fueled fear of sacral energies in their more intense expressions.

These creative energies are what you are attempting to bring forth with the Sacral Lotus Empowerment, and when you do, they can be used in any number of ways within your life. Sacral energy can be used to connect more deeply with people in your life, including a lover if you express this energy sexually. It can be used to help you connect more fully with your sense experience or your environment, whether that's enjoying a glass of fine wine or a beautiful sunset. You might use sacral energy to empower your creativity or look at a difficult work problem in a new way. Or if you're feeling stuck and rigid in your life, the Sacral Lotus will help you find the freshness and inspiration you need to create something new.

Although the second chakra is the anchor for a woman's energy body, this does not mean that being an empowered woman revolves around making the second chakra energies your primary energies. I am not saying that a woman's natural state is desirous, spontaneous, passionate, creative, sexual, and sensual. For some women, these qualities may indeed be the main ways they express their power in the world … and it may be this way for some men, too! Being fully in your power and activating all of your chakras is about discovering and owning the way energy comes through you uniquely. It is *not* about the energies of one particular chakra, even the sacral, being dominant in your personality and awareness. As well, is it not about defining male and female, masculine and feminine in a rigid way. What an empowered sacral chakra does is help you unleash *your* truest nature, *your* unique emanation of energy and awareness into the world. Sacral energies are never about conformity.

Alea was an artist who had hit a major creative block. She had long supported herself through jewelry making and paintings sold in local shops in her seaside town. She now found herself uninspired and unmotivated. Tired of making the same things over and over, she had been trying to experiment with new forms and themes but found herself unexpectedly frozen with self-doubt and lack of ideas. She felt bored and emotionally numb.

Alea began working with the Sacral Lotus on a daily basis. As she activated these energies, she began to acknowledge other shifts that were occurring in her life. In recent years, her sex life with her partner had slowed to almost nothing, and they had never discussed it. In addition, although they had both agreed they did not want children, she now found herself mourning the loss of this possibility. All in all, Alea had many themes related to sexuality and being in a woman's body that were kicking around in her psyche.

Alea continued her daily Sacral Lotus session and began to deal with some of these issues. She and her partner talked about their sex life and decided to take steps to increase their intimacy. She realized she still felt she did not want her own children but wanted to connect more with her young nieces in order to feed her nurturing desires. In addition, Alea began to shift the way she was working, and begin each studio session with an unstructured "free play" time, preceded by activating the Sacral Lotus for just a minute or two. During this time Alea would fingerpaint, doodle, dance around, or do anything that came into her mind, with no judgment, and no thought to end product. Interestingly, the first few times she tried this, she found herself painting different visions of how the Sacral Lotus felt to her. Over time, Alea began developing a vision for a new line of paintings and also started working with ceramics. She felt reinspired and connected to her creativity.

You do not have to be an artist to experience a block. We all draw upon our creativity in some way within our lives, and we all hit phases where we feel uninspired and numb. Whether you are trying to solve a problem at work, redecorate your home, or plan an event, if you are dry of ideas, try the Sacral Lotus to open and free yourself up. Alea's story also points to the deep connection between our level of inspiration and our sense of ourselves as women. It's not a coincidence that she was struggling with issues of sexuality, procreation, and creativity all at once. Working with the Sacral Lotus helped open her up in all three areas.

When You Have Felt This Before

You have felt Sacral Lotus energies whenever you have felt inspired by an idea, by a person, by a work of art, or anything you have connected to that has uplifted you and created a sense of potential. This is what inspiration is, after all—an uplifting sense of new potential. Truly, when the sacral chakra is activated through inspiration it feels like a rising up of energy in your body. You may think of inspiration as felt in your heart, as an upswell of positive emotion, or in your mind, with a burst of sudden ideas, but when you tune in more deeply to inspiration, you will be able to sense the energy rising up from deep in your pelvis. Tapping into memories of past moments of inspiration may be very helpful to you when activating the Sacral Lotus.

Inspiration as muse for creativity is another way you may have experienced the energies of this chakra before. If you are an artist of any type, think of how it feels when a new idea comes to you and you are swept up in the excitement of its evolution. Or perhaps your work evolves as you engage with it, and rather than an idea popping into your head, you find yourself in a magical flow in which you are creating something you could never have conceptualized beforehand. Either way, a burst of creativity is sacral energy. And of course you do not need to be an artist to have experienced this; perhaps it occurs when you are brainstorming new ideas at work with your project team, redecorating your home, or planning a birthday party for your child. Anytime you are caught up in a flow of ideas related to creating something, you are experiencing this aspect of sacral energy.

Another way you may have experienced the energies of this chakra before is in your most powerful sense experiences. When you bite into a delicious piece of chocolate, are awed by a gorgeous ocean view, transported by a beautiful piece of music, or soothed by a quiet walk in the woods, you are in the throes of the sacral. These are moments of union with your senses, when the experience of sensual pleasure induces a feeling of satiation and wholeness. Of course this applies to sexual pleasure and the feeling of oneness with a partner as well. At its best, sexual union encompasses flow, pleasure, spontaneity, and passion, all aspects of the sacral.

If you can relate to any of these energies, jot down your memories of having experienced them, and use them during the activation steps for the Sacral Lotus.

Activation Steps

First review the preparatory steps from the Root Bowl chapter. Settle yourself in a quiet, private space. Prepare the audio file if you are using the online guided recordings, and review any memories of when you have felt this before. Gaze at the Sacral Lotus visual available in the insert for a few centering breaths before beginning.

> *Step 1:* Place your hands over your lower pelvis, hip level and below on your belly, and breathe into your hands for a few centering breaths.

> *Step 2:* Inside your pelvis beneath your hands begin to visualize a large, radiant, amber-colored lotus facing upward, like a large bowl sitting in your lower torso.

Step 3: Take some time to develop this lotus. You can experiment with the size and shape of the petals, and different hues of amber, gold, and orange.

Step 4: The energy of this lotus is fluid, moving, luminous, open, feminine, creative, sensual, and powerful. To connect with the feeling of fluidity, you can sway your body as you visualize if you like. You may keep your hands on your lower belly or move them to rest on your knees or lap.

Step 5: Once you feel connected to the visual of this lotus within your pelvis, begin to imagine roots reaching downward through your tailbone and into the earth, anchoring the lotus.

Step 6: Visualize rays of amber, gold, and orange light radiating upward into the rest of your body and chakras. Imagine it flowing upward out of the top of your head.

Step 7: If you are working with memories of when you have felt sacral energy before, bring them to mind now. Cycle through each one until the associated feeling rises up within you. Imagine this feeling is emanating from your Sacral Lotus and spreading throughout your body as the amber light.

Step 8: Say each of the affirmations associated with this Empowerment one to three times, striving to feel what you are saying as you do:

> I am creative.
> I go with the flow.
> I am a sensual being.
> I am passionate.
> I am inspired.
> I am amazing.

Step 9: Hold this visual for two to three minutes (longer is fine!) When your mind wanders, re-create it in the same order—lotus, roots, upward light. Continue to sway your body if you like. If you feel a particular feeling or energy arise as you do this, relax into that and allow it to guide your vision and experience.

Step 10: Note how you are feeling and take your snapshot memory for fast reference later. Dissolve the visual within you and sit with your eyes closed for a while longer to integrate. Open your eyes and imagine you are seeing the world in a new way.

Now relax and take stock of how you feel. Tune in to your body and notice any sensations. Note your mood and whether it has shifted at all since before you started. Open your awareness to physical and emotional subtleties you might not usually focus on. Don't worry if you don't notice anything, but do take the time to take stock in this way each time you complete an activation. In today's over-stimulated world, most of us have become numb to vibrational shifts, and it may take you some time to sensitize yourself… but it will happen! Keep an open mind, and remember you are engaged in an experiential process.

One unique aspect of the Sacral Lotus (along with one other Empowerment in this book, Feminine Pathway) is that the swaying movement may really help you to connect with the energies you are activating. You may not be able to sway when activating this Empowerment in a particular moment in your day, but do give it a try when you are first practicing activating the Sacral Lotus at home on your own.

When You Are Blocked

One of the primary ways that blocked sacral energy may manifest in you is in the feeling of being stuck. Within daily life, it may manifest as feeling stuck in a situation or being stuck in a particular dynamic with someone. Perhaps you are literally stuck in a meeting and it gives rise to feelings of frustration that prevent you from contributing. Perhaps you are stuck in irritation with your spouse and despite vowing to relate differently, you find yourself coming home and falling into the same old irritated pattern each day. Or you may feel stuck in a larger context, trapped in the routine of your life, weighed down by your responsibilities, numbed and uninspired by the sameness of each day.

Another manifestation of the "stuckness" prevalent when your sacral energies are not active is feeling as if your creativity is blocked. If you're an artist, you may feel as if the muse has left you. Within work or any other endeavors that you're involved in you may feel as if inspiration has left you. When you are trying to solve a problem or think outside the box you feel as if you have hit a wall. Your efforts may feel labored and forced—there is no flow, no momentum or power bringing forth ideas.

Another way a block to this chakra may manifest is as rigidity and an inability to accept change when it arises. For example, say you have plans to go out to dinner with a friend. The date and time have been set for some time, but your friend calls you at the last minute and says she needs to move it because she has been called into work. Rationally, you know this is out of her control, but some part of you clenches up at the change and you find yourself upset with your friend, perhaps anxious and unmoored by the change in your evening. You are unable to accept the change and feel a kind of inner gripping and rigidity. A pattern of rigidity may also express as a need to plan everything to the point of hypercontrol.

Emotional numbness is also a sign of a blocked or weak sacral chakra. Numbness is different than sadness, because when we are numb we can't allow ourselves to feel any emotion, positive or negative. We have a lid on our emotional life or only allow certain emotions, repressing others. The patterns of control and rigidity are applied to our emotional life, and we feel dry and uninspired. This may extend into an inability to experience pleasure, even simple pleasures like enjoying good food or a moving song. Perhaps there is a disconnection from sense experience altogether, with an overemphasis on the mind and mental, rather than sense-based physical, experience.

Sexually this may express as an inability to feel pleasure or connect with a sexual partner in an intimate way. Sex may be robotic and unemotional. Even if you experience physical pleasure, you may disconnect from the emotion or even feel guilt about the pleasure. Sexual shame (and indeed, shame of all forms) is also linked to blocks in the sacral energies. Shame is a feeling of unworthiness, a feeling of being essentially bad, and it often locks us in the patterns of rigidity and numbness related to a blocked sacral chakra.

Using the Sacral Lotus

Once you are comfortable activating the Sacral Lotus through the full process, you can experiment with activating it through the shortcut of the snapshot memory you created in the final step. Flash quickly on both the visual and the feeling from this memory and see if you can bring this energy into a moment in which you need it. At first you may need to do so alone for a couple of minutes in a quiet location, but eventually you will be able to flash upon it instantly to access more of the Sacral Lotus energies when you need them.

Here are some examples of daily situations in which you may want to activate the Sacral Lotus:

- Before or during a break within a work meeting in which you are brainstorming ideas or attempting to look at a problem in a new way.
- To generate ideas for a creative activity such as painting, writing, planning an event or redecorating a room.
- While you are preparing an inspirational or motivational talk for employees at work, a children's sporting team you are coaching, or even your child before a big event in their life.
- When you are having a hard time adapting to a change in your day.
- When you feel trapped or frustrated by circumstances beyond your control—a traffic jam, or meeting that runs long.
- When you feel disconnected from the beauty or sense experience you are in.
- Before an intimate encounter, whether sexual or emotional in nature (or both).

As with all the Empowerments, you may at times want to combine them with each other, doing one first and then the other. The Root Bowl and Sacral Lotus work together particularly well in situations where you recognize that you are being overly controlling. Since this behavior is usually born of anxiety, first activate the Root Bowl to bring forth a feeling of safety and security. Next, activate the Sacral Lotus to generate the energies of fluidity, adaptability, and flow in the moment. Of course, if control issues are not new for you, as with any of the blocks, you may want to look at using the Sacral Chakra for long-term growth.

You may also want to do this Empowerment when you are in a phase of your life in which you feel particularly challenged and unable to access sacral energies. Remember that when you are working with an Empowerment for long-term growth, you commit to activating the Empowerment regularly independent of triggering situations—as with exercise or a meditation routine—in order to build up the associated energies over time in your awareness and energy body.

Here are some examples of when you may want to work with the Sacral Lotus in this way:

- If you are feeling stuck in your life and cannot decide how to change it. You may feel stuck in your job, your relationship, your health, your finances, or all of the above.

- If you feel you are rigid or uptight with others. If you feel this is an expression of anxiety, you may also want to work with the Root Bowl, but in terms of improving your ability to be in the moment and in the flow within social encounters, work with the Sacral Lotus.

- If you feel there is a lid on your emotions, resulting in a kind of emotional dryness or numbness. Of course, if you feel you have repressed emotions related to traumatic events in your life, or are experiencing depression, you may need to pursue mental health counseling. But if you feel the issue is your relationship with your own emotions, and a pattern of blocking them, utilizing the Sacral Lotus for a period of time will help you to open your emotional range. This may in fact be a good counterpart to therapy or counseling on emotional issues.

- If you are about to embark upon a big creative project, consider doing the Sacral Lotus daily for a time, either just before you begin or during the early stages.

- When trying to get pregnant—the initiation of physical creation (along with the Feminine Pathway).

- If you are experiencing a creative block, use the Sacral Lotus to reconnect with your muse.

- If you feel disconnected from your sense experience, trapped in your mind, and in a wholly cerebral relationship with the world. Of course if you feel this is a form of disassociation rooted in trauma, you should pursue mental health support if you have not already done so.

- To ignite or reignite your sex life. However, if sexual difficulties are rooted in sexual trauma, it's important to address other aspects of your sacral chakra and mental health issues first, and to never force sexual activity before you are ready. This topic is covered more in the Sexual Trauma section of this chapter.

- To let go of feelings of shame or unworthiness, particularly shame related to your sexuality or female body.

- Before meeting with a group of women with which you want to deeply connect over feminine issues.

- To connect with the divine feminine and your own feminine power.

Two other key Empowerments in this book involve the sacral chakra—Healing Rays and Feminine Pathway. In the chapters on these Empowerments we will talk more about the sacral chakra's role in aiding healing, supporting us during life transits, and its links to our reproductive cycles and phases.

Women's Energetics: Our Feminine Base

An oft-used metaphor for the latent power of the chakras is that of a snake lying coiled at the base of the spine, the seat of the root chakra. As we begin to work with our chakras, the snake rises up from its coil, most resembling a cobra's rise under the influence of a snake charmer. The snake energy weaves upward, winding through our energy channels and chakras, until it arrives at the crown chakra, at which point it lights up this center of spiritual realization. Sometimes the rising energy is shown as two rising snakes, as in the Greek caduceus symbol used to represent medicine.

While this can be a helpful metaphor for understanding the upward path of energy through the chakras, it is primarily based on the masculine energy body, which is anchored in the root chakra. For women, the Sacral Lotus therefore offers a more accurate visual for our feminine energy body. You might think of a Sacral Lotus bud not yet open as the equivalent of the snake lying coiled. As your sacral opens—into the full flower as in the Sacral Lotus visual—and strong roots develop down through the root chakra, radiant light and energy emanate up through all of the rest of your chakras.

Women's spirituality teachings often talk of womb energy and the creative power available to us because of our connection to procreation. Within energy medicine, our second chakra is linked to our uterus and our ovaries. In this day and age, many women are reluctant to think of their power as rooted in their womb, reproductive organs, or second chakra because it seems to affirm the misogynist view that we are defined by our procreative role, that a woman's value lies in birthing children.

In actuality, praising and embracing the ability to procreate is not what it means for our power to be anchored in our second chakra. The link has more to do with how our journey to power unfolds and the themes that lie at its heart. We don't have to birth children, and neither does having children assure an open and strong second chakra. Instead, our embracing of our power involves fully developing the primary second chakra drives of *connecting to* and *creating in* the world. As we focus on strengthening all the energies of this chakra through the Sacral Lotus, our understanding of ourselves and how we can create the life we want comes forth from these energies. All the energies of the second chakra play a special role in our development—inspiration, creativity, emotion, pleasure, sensuality, and yes, sexuality too.

On a more technical level, the fact that our energy body is anchored in our second chakra has other implications. While the root chakra is about stability and security, the sacral chakra is about flow and movement expressed as both reaching out to connect and in the process of creating. From an energetics perspective, this translates into two prevalent characteristics of women's energy bodies as compared to men's:

- **Women's energy bodies are more centripetal.** Although everyone's energy bodies both attract and emanate energy, ours are in general more absorbent, and receptive, pulling energy in from around us. This energy may be in the form of other's emotions and thoughts, in the form of vibrations from physical surroundings, or in the form of etheric and spiritual input. Depending on how we learn to handle this influx of energetic "data," we might be exceptionally intuitive, suggestible, or just overwhelmed (many of us swing between these). For this reason, we will focus on energetic boundaries, particularly in the Second Skin Empowerment chapter.

- **Women's energy bodies run in cycles and phases.** The sacral chakra is about movement, flow, and change; for women, it manifests as physical and energetic cycles. Just as our physical bodies experience a hormonal cycle every month in our premenopausal years, so our energy bodies flow in time with these. Our energy bodies also shift during pregnancy, postpartum, and menopause. We will discuss all of these shifts in later chapters.

Men also absorb energy from the world around them, and of course men's physical and energy bodies also have phases and cycles. It's a matter of emphasis rather than difference. For women, the most profound personal work often centers on releasing feelings of inferiority, shame, or weakness associated with being in a women's body, so that these differences may be owned as a source of strength and gifts. As women's empowerment has progressed over the last few decades, it has rightly focused on women's access to power in the social, cultural, and political realms. But it is important to note that the success itself has largely involved women succeeding in greater numbers within power structures built by men within patriarchal history. The mantra has been "women can do anything men can do," and certainly this is true. But it has left many women with the feeling that they need to somehow "make up" or compensate for being in a woman's body to "prove" it is not a liability, rather than focusing on developing its inherent and unique strengths and energies. The denigration of women's bodies and many of the energies associated with the sacral chakra—including emotion, which is often seen as weak—has only enforced this tendency.

On a deep level, working with the Sacral Lotus is part of reclaiming your connection to feminine energy as a source of power. It has nothing to do with expressing yourself only through sacral energies, or in defining yourself in terms of your procreative role. It has everything to do with surfacing and letting go of any feelings of being "less than" that you still harbor as a woman. It is about tuning in to who you are as an individual, and manifesting a life founded on happiness and empowerment rooted in this knowledge. This is a right that should be afforded to all of us, men and women, and as the shifts in our society continue, we will have more freedom to do so.

Sexual Trauma Healing:
Releasing Shame, Allowing Pleasure

Sexual abuse and assault are about power. They are about domination, disempowerment, and manipulation. For an abuser or assaulter, power and sex have become dysfunctionally entwined, and part of the damage for sexual trauma survivors is that society often forces this dysfunction on them as well. Survivors receive countless victim-blaming messages from all around them, telling them that their own sexuality and sexual energy is at fault, and/or that they are weak. Their own sexual energy and feelings of disempowerment become linked, and they are made to feel shame … shame becomes linked to having a female body. Body hatred, disempowerment, and the feeling that being female is a liability are often intensified.

While this doesn't play out in the same way for every woman, usually there are several areas of the sacral chakra that are blocked in some way. And because of the sacral chakra's centrality in the feminine energy body, this affects their entire energy body. If you feel this is true for you, a big part of your healing is releasing shame and the belief that your own sexual energy is a liability and weakness. One way this can express itself is an internal repression of the sacral energies. Think about each of the main sacral energies we have discussed in this chapter, apart from sexuality for now—inspiration, creativity, sensuality, fluidity, and emotion. Which of these do you feel are strong in you, and which are weak? Have you disconnected from any of these energies because they don't feel safe to you? If so, then working with both the Root Bowl and Sacral Lotus for a period of time may be very beneficial. You can cultivate the sense of safety you need with Root Bowl followed by empowering your weaker sacral energies through the Sacral Lotus.

Just the practice of having your hands on your lower belly and visualizing a beautiful lotus in your pelvis is in and of itself healing. It will begin to unwind the layers of conditioning around this area of your body, and of sacral energies being bad or shameful. Try to cultivate a new connection with this part of your body, a new sense of love and appreciation.

Of course, the sacral center is linked to sexuality, an area greatly effected for most sexual trauma survivors. Some survivors cannot engage in sexual relations at all, while others can but do not relate to it as a source of pleasure or intimacy. Working through sexual issues of this nature often requires counseling, especially if sexual activity triggers flashbacks or disassociation. Apart from that, working with the Sacral Lotus can be a powerful aid. Experiment with activating the Sacral Lotus for a period of time before engaging in some pleasurable sense-based experience that is *not* sexual in nature— listening to music, visiting an art gallery, taking a candlelit bath, or even eating your favorite food. As you become more comfortable with sensual pleasure *apart* from sex, and the energies of the Sacral Lotus increase in your energy body, with time this will begin to carry over into your relationship with sex itself.

Some sexual trauma survivors act out feelings of unworthiness or shame by engaging in risky sexual behavior or by engaging in sexual encounters that mirror or copy the ways they were abused or assaulted. If this is true for you, consider taking a break from sexual activity for a period of time that you feel is realistic, and focus on the Sacral Lotus daily during that time. Seek to establish a healthy link between your sacral energies, your body, and your psyche.

However, having an empowered sacral chakra and feminine energy body does not require being sexually active. On the contrary, in some historical women's spiritual traditions, the female healers and seers were celibate by choice, partly because this meant that their sacral energies could be channeled into their work. Similarly, a strong sacral has nothing to do with birthing children, as there are many other ways we manifest our creative energies in the world. What is most essential is that you decide what is right for you in relation to your sexuality and your sacral energies in general, and that you allow this to change over time.

From an energetics perspective, women who experience sexual trauma often feel double-victimized—first through the actual abuse or assault, and then again through the disconnection from their own sacral energies that frequently results. An important part of healing is recognizing the need to heal on both levels. Seek the support you need to heal from the physical and psychological trauma. Then focus for a time on reestablishing your link to your sacral chakra energies. Cultivate a healthy, loving relationship with your own body and sacral energies, and begin to embrace being a woman as a source of strength and power. Working with the other Empowerments in this book will continue your evolution in this regard.

Emily had scheduled energy work sessions because she had been date-raped in college and never acknowledged it. She had read about my sexual trauma energy work and wanted to explore it, as she felt perhaps her experience was affecting her ability to find a healthy relationship. The first thing I noticed about Emily was that she apologized even when there was no need—she did so first for being late (she wasn't), second for not sending me more pre-session background information (it was optional), and third for having slight laryngitis (I couldn't tell).

As we talked about what had happened to her, it was clear Emily blamed herself. She had willingly gone with her assaulter to his dorm room, and they had begun to kiss. As he started to push things further, she said no. When he didn't comply, she tried to push him away. This went on for some time, until she tried to get away and leave the room. At that point, he forced himself on her, and she went limp to get it over with. When she told a friend afterward what had happened, she was sympathetic and said, "What a jerk," but did not seem to think it was anything unusual and relayed a similar incident that she had experienced. This normalized the encounter for Emily, who did not think of it as assault and blamed herself. She pushed the memory away and never spoke of it again.

I encouraged Emily to look into counseling services for sexual assault and advised her on good reading material and online resources that would help her to understand date rape and her responses. Then we began to work gently with the Sacral Lotus and the theme of shame/self-blame. I asked Emily to activate the Sacral Lotus each day for a week and to try to activate it quickly within her day whenever she realized she had just said "I'm sorry" for something that was not really her fault or even a problem.

Emily reported back the next week that she had not been able to do the second exercise completely, because she had discovered she apologized so frequently and habitually it would have been impossible. She realized she felt sorry and at fault all the time. In fact, she realized this pattern had been present before her assault and was connected to feelings of unworthiness and perfectionism developed in childhood, but that it had become more pronounced after her assault.

She continued to work with the Sacral Lotus regularly, especially when she felt herself feeling guilty or apologetic. Over time, she released the shame she had felt over her assault, and told her mother and a trusted friend what had happened. Being able to share her story in this way empowered her and contributed to her healing. As she shifted out of the habit of constantly feeling at fault and owned her right to be in the world on her own terms, she began to live from a more empowered place within herself.

Emily's story is all too common and reflected in many other settings. Even if you have not experienced an explicit sexual assault, chances are you have experienced sexual harassment or discomfort at some point in your life that left you with feelings of shame or self-blame. Even without these experiences, women are often socialized to believe they are responsible for everything that happens to and around them, and it can show itself in the tendency to apologize that Emily exhibited. Working with the Sacral Lotus can aid you in releasing these feelings and help you stake your claim to your rightful place in the world as a woman who expects respect.

THREE
Navel Fire:
Your Personal Power

Related Chakras: Your navel, or third, chakra

Energies: Sense of self, personal power, willpower, determination, confidence, discipline, endurance, organization, information processing, execution, detachment, objectivity

Use For: Passivity, insecurity, lack of confidence, procrastination, lack of motivation, obstacles, lack of focus, hyperactivity, whenever you need to empower your ability to lead, present, or act

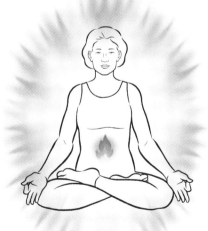

When we say someone has a fire in their belly, we mean they are driven and able to push through any obstacle to achieve their goal. This is one expression of navel chakra energies, and it is what the Navel Fire activates. When your Navel Fire is lit, you feel you can accomplish what you've set your mind to and overcome any challenge. You are focused and motivated, determined and organized. You have a plan and the will and concentration to execute it.

The energies of the navel chakra are the center point from which we interact with the world. It is the nexus of our sense of self in the world—us in relation to the world. It therefore has a lot to do with our ability to act. What do we feel capable of doing "out there," outside of ourselves? While the root and sacral chakras are about our relationship to our body and emotions, and our senses of security and connection, the navel is then about the next step, the outward facing step—our intent, action, and impact.

On the level of our psyche, navel chakra energies reflect our self-confidence and self-esteem—do we believe we can act effectively in the world? On the level of skill, these energies manifest as our ability to harness our mental energy in an effective way—do we have the focus, determination, organizational ability, and endurance to accomplish what we've set out to do? Working with the Navel Fire will help you on both fronts. It will help you to surface and 'burn' away limiting self-beliefs that hold you back, and it will also help you to increase your mental focus and clarity, as well as activate your will and endurance. For women, an important part of working with the Navel Fire is clearing any limiting beliefs we have internalized about our ability or right to act in the world, or in certain arenas of the world.

Because the navel chakra is the center of our energy in relation to the world, it's defined by a constant flow of give and take. Ideally, there is a balance between receptivity and assertiveness—our ability to *absorb* the world and our ability to *act* in it. But if we are out of balance, this can become passivity or aggression, or an erratic swing between the two (passive-aggressive behavior.) An effective and empowered navel chakra is about balance, a balance between our ability to observe and make sense of the world, and our ability to take action and put our stamp on it.

The metaphor of a fire is very helpful for understanding this balance. When you are trying to start a fire from a spark or ember, you need to provide just the right amount of air to ignite it, bursting into flame. No matter if you fan or blow on it or use a bellows, the right amount of air is crucial—enough for the ember to spark but not so much that the flame blows out before it catches or the ember extinguishes. In the same way, working with your Navel Fire is about balance. A raging, uncontrolled flame is not what you are after—that just generates energies of dominance, aggression, and destruction. Neither do you want a weak, tenuous flame, because then you aren't claiming the space you need and deserve in the world. A balanced, healthy, centered heat and expression of power is what we need.

Our navel chakra is also very much about boundaries, the lines we draw between ourselves and others. This means boundaries in terms of our ability to say no (breaking out of people-pleasing), boundaries in terms of insisting upon the respectful treatment we deserve, and energetic boundaries—our ability to create an energetic filter that screens the energies we allow into our energy body from other people and the world around us. In this chapter we will mostly talk about boundaries in terms of the first two types, but we will talk about energetic boundaries in the Second Skin Empowerment chapter.

The Navel Fire is also a great Empowerment for clearing out energies from our physical body and psyche that are unhealthy for us, like an energy detox. We can burn away negative emotions or tension we have picked up from people around us, or from an environment we have been in. This process has a clarifying and centering effect, disintegrating any force within us that has pulled us off balance. It centers us back into our power.

Shanea was in her midthirties and frustrated in her current job search. While she had constantly earned praise in her work as a web developer, acknowledged as a hard worker and good team member, it had not resulted in a promotion. She had watched coworkers around her (including women) move ahead. She felt she was undervalued, viewed as "reliable Shanea" but never given new opportunities at her firm. She had decided to look for a new job and had landed a couple of interviews through a recruiter but had been so nervous in both that she had not performed well and had not been offered either job.

Shanea was very drawn to the law of attraction and positive thinking teachings. She had created many vision boards and other Empowerments for helping her to achieve her goals. She also had read many books about women in business and recognized some patterns of capitulating and people-pleasing that were not serving her. She felt these books and Empowerments had helped her to clarify her intent and communication, but she was beginning to blame herself for not having yet achieved what she wanted. She wondered if she wasn't trying hard enough, wasn't good enough, was holding herself back, or was really too comfortable or even lazy. She wondered if she was engaging in self-sabotage or not performing her daily affirmations correctly. She was filled with self-doubt, uncertainty, and feelings of unworthiness.

In our first session I guided Shanea through activating her Navel Fire, and we focused on each of her doubts in turn, imagining them as dark blocks around her navel and solar plexus area. We visualized her Navel Fire expanding and burning these doubts to ash, like a candle would burn slips of paper. I then asked Shanea to focus on three recent accomplishments at her current job, which we imagined as balls of light in her belly, brightening her Navel Fire even more and emanating light outward from her being. Finally, I asked Shanea to imagine herself in confident conversations with her current boss, the recruiter, and in an imaginary interview, one after the other, each with her Navel Fire lit and emanating light and power outward throughout each exchange.

I suggested that following the session Shanea put away her vision boards and goal-based affirmations for now and instead repeat the second half of the exercise we had done together every day: activating her Navel Fire, focusing on recent successes, and imagining herself emanating the light of these successes and her Navel Fire outward while in confident exchanges with her boss, recruiter, and future interviewers. I also suggested that she try to take a minute-long break if possible during her day whenever she felt self-doubt or people-pleasing patterns arise, and imagine burning up that feeling or tendency as a block in her belly with her Navel Fire.

Shanea began to assert herself more at work. She made a point of noticing and magnifying her successes and communicating them to others when appropriate. She also asked the recruiter for more specific feedback from her prior interviews, and the information she received helped her to modify her resume to better highlight her achievements. She practiced communicating these achievements in an interview setting and eventually landed a new interview. Before her interview, Shanea activated her Navel Fire, and again reminded herself of her past accomplishments. She felt much less nervous in the interview, and received the job offer she wanted. Much to her surprise, her current boss was genuinely upset when Shanea told her she was leaving and made a counteroffer. Shanea decided to make a fresh start and move to the new company. She continued to work with themes related to owning her power and confidence and has continued to succeed in her work since that time.

Shanea's experience highlights one of the most important ways we build our navel energies and the associated self-confidence and personal power—by focusing on accomplishments we have *already* achieved. Again, a fire metaphor is very apropos—a fire grows bigger when you provide it more fuel, and highlighting past accomplishments and successes is fuel for your Navel Fire. It is easy when doing personal development or aspirational work to get stuck in our deficiencies—all the goals we haven't yet achieved, or all the ways we are doing something "wrong." We can get stuck in this negative frame of mind, which is like throwing a wet blanket over our fire.

Aspirations and goals are important, and setting ambitious ones can be a crucial part of developing your personal power in the world. But if you find you have become focused on your failure to achieve a goal and are beset by doubts and self-criticism, then allow yourself to burn that away and focus instead on the fuel of past successes while building your Navel Fire. Of course, success is also about focus and hard work; and in this case Shanea kept at it, getting feedback from her recruiter, modifying her resume, and honing her interview skills. In the end it was the combination of this diligence along with her inner shifts that enabled her to achieve this step and bring about lasting changes.

When You Have Felt This Before

Shanea's story highlights one of the main times you have felt the energy of the Navel Fire before—whenever you have achieved something and truly felt proud of yourself. If you have difficulty acknowledging your own accomplishments, I encourage you to sit down and recapitulate your life, focusing on your moments of achievement. These do not have to be successes acknowledged by others—the important thing is that in the moment you felt you had accomplished something. The aftermath of your accomplishment is also not relevant in this case (e.g., if you are proud of the garden you created at your last home but know that the garden was removed by the home's current residents). What's important is that in the moment the garden was completed, you felt proud of it.

Any activity in which you feel confident of your ability is also a time in which your navel chakra is strong. Perhaps you are confident in work, school, parenting, or some other worldly arena that is acknowledged by others. Don't just look there, however—think in broader terms. Do you have a hobby in which you feel sure of yourself? A sport or exercise regimen? Do you feel confident when baking, or listening to a friend's problems, or hiking up a mountain? Focus on moments when you are free of self-doubt or uncertainty.

Another expression of Navel Fire that you may have felt before is determination. Think of a time in your life in which you have felt very determined, or an activity in which you've had to draw upon this. There is a very quick way to tap into this particular expression of navel energy that you can do right now. Ask yourself: How many push-ups or sit-ups or leg lifts (or similar) do I think I can realistically do? Come up with a number, and then give it a try—right now. When you reach your goal, or at whatever point you want to quit, challenge yourself to do just two or three more (don't hurt yourself… that's not the point of this exercise)! In those few moments in which you override your desire to quit and push on, you are accessing the determination side of your navel chakra. After you stop, take a moment to remember what it felt like in those moments, the feeling of determination in your body.

As with all the chakras, just because determination is an example of drawing upon your navel chakra, this does not mean you will necessarily feel it in your belly. You may feel it somewhere else or as a whole-body sensation. At the level of your energy body, however, this energy is centered in your belly area, and you can draw upon this memory when working to explicitly activate your Navel Fire.

Our navel chakra energy is not just about feeling, it is also about precision in the form of organization and efficiency. If you are someone who can break down a project into smaller steps and map a specific path to completion, this is another example you can draw upon when activating your Navel Fire. If you are good at organizing others or a space—even your closet or cupboards—think about the clarity of mind you experience while doing so. If you are good at making sense out of data, processing information in a useful way, then draw upon the mental state and focus you enter into while engaged in this. All of these are also expressions of Navel Fire in its targeted, active emanation.

Another example of this aspect of navel chakra energies is the ability to step back from a situation and assess it objectively (or as objectively as possible). The ability to cut through emotions and attachments, consider both sides of an issue or conflict, or pull back and see the big picture is linked to the balanced, more abstract emanation of navel chakra energies. If you are good at mediating disputes, listening to a friend's problem and helping her see it in a new way, or guiding a group through problem-solving to reach a strategic objective, these are also examples you may want to draw upon.

Activation Steps

As always, find a quiet, private space when you are first learning to activate your Navel Fire. Prepare the audio file and have your When You Have Felt This Before references handy. You may also want to have a list of self-doubts or self-limiting beliefs that you have identified as active for you.

Gaze at the Navel Fire picture for a minute to familiarize yourself with it. You can also light a candle and place it in front of you. Some people find it helpful to imagine a candle flame mirrored in their navel while they are first working to activate this Empowerment.

> *Step 1:* Establish your seat and place your hands just below your navel. Take a few deep centering breaths, focusing on expanding your belly just under your hands as you do so, like a balloon expanding and contracting with each breath.

Step 2: You may keep your hands on your stomach if you like or rest them in your lap. Begin to visualize a brilliant yellow flame just under your navel, like a large candle flame glowing warm and bright. If you are using an actual lit candle, open your eyes and gaze at this flame, imagining it mirrored below your own navel.

Step 3: Spend some time breathing into this flame, feel your belly continue to rise and fall with your breath, and imagine that your breath is fueling this flame, it slowly growing brighter and brighter, spreading heat throughout your body.

Step 4: If you have specific self-doubts or insecurities currently present in your life, briefly bring each one to mind and imagine it is a dark bit of matter in your belly area. Then imagine that your Navel Fire lights this piece of matter on fire, and it dissolves into ash and then disappears completely. Repeat this for each doubt or insecurity you are working with.

Step 5: Now bring to mind your moments of success, or other When You Have Felt This Before memories, one by one. Recall the feeling of these moments, and imagine they are fueling your Navel Fire, triggering it to burn brighter and warmer. Feel this heat expanding throughout your entire body.

Step 6: Cultivate a feeling of this fire being the center of your confidence, of it radiating off of you in waves. Cultivate the feeling of laser-like focus and determination. Because it's a consolidated energy, some people find that placing their hands in fists really helps to fuel this sense of power and focus and centeredness.

Step 7: Imagine this confidence, this power, this heat is radiating out in all directions from you. You have a sphere of yellow-orange light all the way around you, emanating in every direction, centered in your Navel Fire.

Step 8: Feeling this heat and power, say each of the associated affirmations:
I am powerful.
I am confident.
I am organized.
I am determined.

I am focused.

I am centered.

Step 9: Hold this visual and feeling for as long as you like. Take your "snapshot" of this state to access quickly when you need it. When you are ready, let go of the visual and open your eyes.

This Empowerment is often one that triggers physical sensations, especially a warmth or a tingle in your belly. Not everyone feels this, and it is not a problem if you do not. But if you do, you can focus on this heat or tingle as part of your activation steps. Include it in your snapshot and see if you can cultivate this feeling whenever you need to activate this Empowerment in your day.

When You Are Blocked

One way to identify blocks to your navel chakra is to think in terms of your Navel Fire burning too low or too high. If it is low, your light is dimmed in the world. You may feel invisible to some or all of the people in your life, or unacknowledged. You may be passive, holding back from saying what you really feel or want. You may feel taken for granted or be stuck in patterns of people pleasing. You may feel as if you take on others' emotions, or that others take their negative emotions out on you.

On the other hand, if the flame of your Navel Fire is too high and uncontrolled, you may be bullish and domineering. You may steamroll over people or engage in hypercontrolling and manipulative behavior. You may engage in conflict a lot or be quick to anger. Your energy may be too intense for others, or frenetic. You may be hyperactive, unfocused, or unable to keep yourself moving in one direction, toward one goal. You may not be able to receive feedback or tune in to what others have to say to you.

Most of us swing a bit between expressions of these two, between passivity and aggression. Or we may be one way in relationships, but another in work, or differ between types of relationships, e.g., passive in romantic relationships but domineering as a parent. Often there are familiar power dynamics from our childhood that play out in our adult life through navel chakra issues. Identifying how you can more fully own your personal power is about figuring out where and in what way you are out of balance in terms of your power dynamics with others.

Energetically, this balance also has to do with the flow of energies between our lower three chakras. Optimally, our root chakra provides the sense of safety and foundation for energy to flow upward from it to our sacral chakra. Our empowered sacral is then able to flow unconstrained, providing us with inspiration and a desire to connect with the world. The navel chakra is then fueled by both energies to have its expression in a balanced, focused power. But when the lower two chakras are not strong, there is often a gripping in our navel chakra. We try to self-generate all of our own power rather than feel fueled by our root and sacral energies. Our navel is flying solo with no support or consistent power source. This is draining and exhausting, and often expresses itself in patterns of swinging between low and high flames— passive and aggressive behaviors.

A balanced Navel Fire lights up as a sense of power coming *through* us, not *from* us. When our Navel Fire is strong, we don't feel like an island, self-generating all of our own power. We don't feel like we have to control everyone or let everyone control us in order to feel okay. We can give and take and move naturally between the two, centered in our strong sense of self. We can handle "hits" to our being—those moments when someone says something hurtful or tries to dim our light—without it really getting to us. We are lit from within, and no one can take that from us.

Using the Navel Fire

Because of the tendency to swing in our navel chakra energies from too weak to too strong, from passive or people-pleasing to aggressive or off-putting, it's helpful to think of both kinds of situations in your day in which you may want to use the Navel Fire. There are times you may need to stoke the fire, and times you need to contain and focus it.

Here are examples of times you may want to focus on building and strengthening your Navel Fire:

- Before or during exercise, to draw upon your maximum determination.

- To clear your energy field of negative energy or emotions you feel you have picked up from people around you or an environment. We will talk more about this in the Second Skin chapter.

- When you need to stand up for yourself. You may activate this Empowerment before a meeting or encounter with someone who you know may bully you or make you feel insecure.

- Before heading into an interview, presentation, big meeting, sporting event, or any event in which you need to project your competence and ability.

- Before and during a physical or mental challenge—for example, a triathlon or big test—in which you especially need to draw upon your determination and endurance.

- When you are feeling scattered or disorganized, or anytime you are about to embark upon an endeavor requiring focus and organizational abilities.

Here are some examples of when you might need to contain or calm your Navel Fire. You will do this in the same way—it is still an activation—but your intention is more centered on *focusing* your power, rather than increasing it.

- When you feel anger arising or just after an angry confrontation. You may eventually shift into the Heart Star (covered in the next chapter), but often during or after feeling angry, we first need to center our navel energies before we can work with the heart.

- When you feel yourself becoming overly controlling or domineering, or after you realize you have been this way. Again, you may find it helpful to activate other Empowerments too, depending on what you feel are the root causes of this tendency; for example, the Root Bowl if it is fear-based.

- When you are hyperactive or frenzied—mentally, physically, or both.

- When gripped by the desire to engage in some activity you know will not be healthy for you. This could be anything from binge eating or drinking, to calling an ex whom you know you are better off without. This isn't a substitute for any long-term therapeutic or healing work you may need to do on the issue, but if you are already engaged in such work, using the Navel Fire in the moment will help you to focus your energies and harness the willpower needed to overcome the urge in the moment.

You may want to work with the Navel Fire daily for a time when you are working to break through patterns of disempowerment, insecurity, or lack of confidence. If you have never really felt like you have been in your power or are working toward shifting your life situation or power dynamics, you'll want to increase the energies associated with the Navel Fire and enable this fiery energy to burn through your old patterns and limiting self-beliefs. Working with the Navel Fire in this way evokes the story of the phoenix (think Fawkes if you are a Harry Potter fan), who burns to dissolution every so often and then is reborn from the ash with a renewed power and wisdom. When you use the Navel Fire for a phase of personal growth in this way, you are generating a mini version of the Phoenix cycle for yourself.

Here are some examples of life situations or long-term patterns you may want to use the Navel Fire every day for:

- If you feel as if you have never truly asserted your power and taken control of your life. You may feel as if you have been swept up by life, never making your own decisions, or you may feel as if you have lived out others' expectations of you.

- If you feel your ability to express your power and live your life has been suppressed by outside forces, whether by individuals in your life, or through institutional or cultural gender, racial, religious, or sexual preference discrimination. Empowering yourself through the Navel Fire will not magically put an end to these forces, of course, but it will enable you to strategize how you might better fight against or change them.

- When undergoing treatment for cancer or healing from a debilitating illness or injury. You may want to combine it with Healing Rays (chapter 10). The Navel Fire will help you to access the determination and endurance you need, while the Healing Rays will help you to increase your self-healing and self-soothing abilities.

- When facing an obstacle or opposition to a long-standing goal.
- When you are working to let go of Power Myths (covered in the next section) and ready to reframe your perception of your own power.
- If you suspect you have difficult thinking in a linear, organized manner.
- When working to break through a long-standing fear or phobia through counseling or other treatments.

Jean was in her midforties and had built a successful business from scratch by herself. Growing up, she had witnessed her mother be repeatedly physically abused by her father until he finally left the family when she was twelve years old. They had very little contact with him after that, and he did not contribute money for the care of her and her younger brother, leaving the family in desperate financial straits. Jean grew up determined to never be vulnerable or poor like her mother. She worked her way through night school as a temporary receptionist and eventually started her own temporary hiring firm, which had grown to three cities and more than fifty employees.

When we began working together, Jean had just gone through a painful divorce and was struggling to relate to her thirteen-year-old son, who had opted to live with his father. She felt angry and beaten down at the same time. She admitted to having struggled with angry outbursts her whole life and had a history of altercations with employees, neighbors, her husband, and son. Although never physical, any perceived slight could trigger these outbursts; once it happened, she would usually go for the jugular and say whatever would hurt the other person the most. In fact, she had just been ordered into anger management classes by a judge due to a case brought against her by a neighbor for verbal harassment (the dispute had started with her complaining about noise but escalated to a highly charged altercation over which the police had been called by another neighbor). Jean had been taking power yoga classes for several years, and at the advice of her yoga teacher had decided to try some chakra work to complement the anger management course.

In our first session, it was hard to reconcile all of this information with the heartbroken, beaten-down woman I was speaking with. Jean believed her anger was ruining her life, and she feared she had inherited this from her father and there was nothing she could do to change. In her anger management class, Jean was learning how to recognize the physical signs in her body of her anger triggering as well as breathing exercises to try to calm herself down when it did. I taught her the Navel Fire Empowerment and suggested she combine it with her breathing Empowerments, imagining that her breath was stabilizing and strengthening her self-control and center in the form of a steady, calm flame. We practiced this by working with a memory of her last angry altercation, feeling the angry energy dispersed throughout her body consolidating into this steady, warm flame in her navel chakra. I also asked her to try the Navel Fire daily for ten minutes, imagining each of her current self-doubts and anxieties were burning in the fire generated.

With time, Jean began to see the swinging pattern of her navel chakra energies in relation to others as well as the pattern's roots. She realized she needed to feel in control and authority in every interaction and could actually feel the gripping in her navel chakra area that accompanied it. If anyone or a situation threatened this feeling of control or authority, she could feel how her navel chakra energies went into overdrive, putting up walls, and fighting against the "threat" through anger. She could also feel how this exhausted and depleted her, leaving her feeling downtrodden and hopeless— the other end of the navel chakra spectrum she was swinging on. She recognized the roots of both ends of this spectrum in the vow she had made as a teenager to never be vulnerable or weak.

As Jean began to work through her issues on a deeper level, we began to also work with the Root Bowl and Sacral Lotus. We worked to create a flow of upward energy from these chakras to fuel her Navel Fire instead of what she had been doing—feeling as though she had to self-generate all of her power. We continued to work with the Navel Fire as a means to burn away old self-beliefs and to center and stabilize her sense of power in relation to others. She began to feel a more organic give-and-take flow of power between herself and others, and she was able to better receive and process criticism or negativity directed her way. As she changed, Jean was able to heal her relationship with her son and stop the destructive angry outbursts that had plagued her in all areas of her life.

Anger is just one of the ways a navel chakra imbalance can express, and of course other chakra blocks may be linked to anger issues. Often there is deep fear, shame, and/or hurt underlying anger, such that work on the root, sacral, and heart are needed. But beginning by stabilizing the Navel Fire and using this energy to center and gain self-control when anger begins to trigger can help you to see the power dynamics at work and the ways you may be defending against feeling vulnerable. It will also empower your sense that you can change and help you to release (that is, burn away) old self-beliefs.

Jean's story also underscores how exhausting it can be to have a hyper-reliance on the navel chakra as an attempt to stem off vulnerability. She had used her personal power well in terms of building a successful business, but because she was constantly self-generating this power without a sense of the underlying security and inspiration from her root and sacral energies supporting her, she frequently felt depleted and alone. Those feelings in turn magnified her tendency to fly off the handle in anger at the slightest provocation. We will work more on the flow between chakras in the Feminine Pathway chapter.

Women's Energetics: Myths of Power

The focal points for the lower three chakras vary the most between energy mappings from different cultures and traditions. I have chosen the placements I have because they are the most helpful for women based on our overall energy system. In chakra mappings that have fewer than seven chakras, the root and sacral are often merged into one lower chakra, and/or the sacral and navel may be merged as well. For women, distinguishing the sacral chakra and working with it low in the pelvic bowl centered at the cervix—the literal doorway to life—is essential to connecting to our primordial creative energy. Distinguishing this from our root chakra, our basic connection to our physical body and security in the material world, is critical: the two energies are very different, and we need them both.

Another common difference is that in some seven-chakra mappings, the focal point for the third chakra is higher (in the solar plexus just below the sternum) instead of just below the navel as we are using for the Navel Fire. In chakra mappings with more than seven chakras, usually the navel and solar plexus are considered separate chakras. In the mapping I am using, the third chakra is still considered linked to the entire stomach area above it; it encompasses the solar plexus area. Only the primary focal point differs: for the Navel Fire, this location just below the navel is a key area for many women. In Eastern-based martial arts and Chinese medicine, this area corresponds to the main nexus for the *hara* or *dan tian*, the centers for personal power, and in particular emanating personal power into the world.

Discovering and developing this kind of power, a personal power that we can emanate and wield in the world, is so important for women right now. Our sacral chakra in the system we are using represents our *inner* power, our connection to our womanhood and the creation energies intrinsic to it, which have been historically devalued and even demonized. Our navel chakra represents our *outer* power—our power in relation to the world, which was historically forbidden to us. As women in today's world, we are working to reclaim and understand both our inner and outer power. Distinguishing these two chakras and their corresponding energies is the most helpful way to energize both. I also work with the solar plexus as an energy center, especially with men, but I have found it is more useful when working with issues of identity as opposed to power.

Most women still have a complicated relationship to worldly power. Much of our conditioning still encourages us not to want or wield it. For these reasons, much of the work that women need to do when working to cultivate our Navel Fire involves identifying and releasing what I call Myths of Power. These are incorrect and limiting beliefs we may be holding, consciously or unconsciously, that prevent us from fully owning our power. Below are some of the most common Myths of Power for women. As you read them, I recommend thinking about how each myth might be functioning under the surface of your life. You can use the Navel Fire to burn away the myths and replace them with truths.

Myth 1: Powerful or assertive women are unlikable. If I claim power in the world or aggressively express myself, I will be unliked/unloved.

This is a myth born of fear—that assertive, strong women will shake the status quo. Women have the right to claim power, manifest as many variations in personality as men, and express themselves in as many ways. True relationships are based on mutual respect and equality. You deserve these kinds of relationships, not ones based on suppression of what you want or think, or on pleasing others.

Truth: If I stand in the world in my power, I will attract people into my life who appreciate me as a I truly am, and I will have relationships based on mutual respect and support.

Myth 2: Men are naturally stable, strong, and powerful, while women are naturally creative, receptive, and nurturing.

We all contain all of these energies. Archetypal male energies are stable, strong, and powerful, and these reflect the strongest aspects of the root chakra. Archetypal female energies are creative, receptive, and nurturing, and these reflect the strongest aspects of the sacral chakra. But we are all composed of all of these. That men's energy bodies are rooted in their root chakras, and women's in their sacral does not mean that men *only* reflect energies of the root while women *only* reflect energies of the sacral. It means that the source of our power and the nature of our personal growth trajectories are intrinsically tied to these chakras. But we are holistic beings; we all need to develop all sides of ourselves. The division of energies and traits along these lines has historically been an excuse to exclude women from authority and external power.

Truth: I am stable, strong, powerful, creative, receptive, nurturing, and many other things. I am a whole being, unique and unto myself. I claim my right to be all of this and more.

Myth 3: Power is evil and corrupt. If I claim it, I will eventually become that way too.

Power itself just is; its use can be for good or evil. Hitler was powerful; so was Rosa Parks. Some people use their power for good, and others do not. Some wield their power loudly, and others do so quietly. I find many women, especially those who have experienced abuse or discrimination at the hands of powerful individuals or organizations, deny themselves power as a kind of rebellion, but all too often they are the ones hurt the most, and others are denied the benefit of their voice and gifts.

Truth: I will use my power how I wish, loudly or quietly, for the good of others or myself. Power is choice.

Myth 4: Power is not spiritual.

Sometimes this myth is rooted in the monastic ideal that removing oneself from the world, or living in it while keeping oneself detached, is spiritually superior. Or sometimes it is based in the idea of 'turning the other cheek', and interpreting this to mean never engaging in conflict or asserting authority of any type. But spiritual awakening, and spiritual action in the world, requires power—a power born of compassion and light. It is not antispiritual to act in this world according to your beliefs.

Truth: We are all agents of power, as cocreators of this world, and spirituality is based on an owning of this.

Myth 5: My power is limited, and if I use too much of it, I will run out.

Ultimately power comes through us, not from us. We are a conduit for it, and working with your Navel Fire, and the other Empowerments in this book, is a way of opening yourself to the unlimited source that is available to you. This doesn't mean you won't get tired—physically, emotionally, or energetically. But this is not permanent—rejuvenation is simply a matter of taking the time to refuel on all levels. You will never run out once you have discovered this, and your capacity to access and hold more will increase throughout your life.

Truth: I am a conduit for unlimited power.

Sexual Trauma Healing: Reclaiming Your Inner Fire

For sexual trauma survivors, many of the Myths of Power are magnified. But there is an additional myth that is often the most destructive: the myth that someone can take your power. Specifically:

Myth 6: My abuser or assaulter took my personal power.

No. No one can take your personal power. They can cause you pain. They can wound you. They may limit your access to organizational power. But they cannot truly take your inner fire from you. Your access to this power is a birthright. Pain can subside, wounds can heal, and you can fight limits placed upon you from the outside—you can reclaim your inner fire.

You may also feel like your abuser(s) or assaulter(s) have taken something from you and still have it. But no one can do this. Anything you feel they may have taken—your sense of worthiness, your ability to trust, your voice—is still accessible to you. As you progress on your healing journey, you will recover access to it within yourself. Your abuser/assaulter has nothing of yours. You do not need to reclaim anything from them. You are done with them.

Truth: My abuser(s)/assaulter(s) abused power to hurt and wound me. But I can heal. They took nothing from me, and have nothing of mine that I need to get back. I am done with them.

Reinforcing this truth is an essential part of the sexual trauma healing journey. Saying you are done with your assaulter(s)/abuser(s) does not mean that you do not pursue justice, not confront them, or tell your story to others. It simply means that you let go of the idea that you need something back from your abuser or assaulter in order to heal. Often there is a holding on to this idea in various forms. It might be that you feel you need them to acknowledge what they did to you, or that you need others to do so. Or you may feel that you need some sign of remorse, or some sign that they are suffering for what they did. But if you wait for any of that, you may wait forever; while you do, your abuser/assaulter is still in control of where you are in your healing process.

So, let that go. This is what it means to say, "I am done with them." You do not need to get your power or anything else *back from* them. It is all inside you, and you need to work on reestablishing your own connection to it. Doing this does not prevent you from pursuing justice or doing whatever else you need to do to fight against your abuser or assaulter, or to fight for social change. This is what the Navel Fire—and all the Empowerments in this book—are meant to help you with.

The other common blocks related to the navel chakra that we have already covered are also often magnified for sexual trauma survivors. You may feel you have ceded all your power to others and become passive or timid, a habituation of the disempowerment you experienced with your abuser or assaulter. If so, you will want to work with the Navel Fire in a fiery way, burning up your fears or feelings of unworthiness and building up your "flame" of assertiveness, confidence, and self-possession. Perhaps you vowed never to be vulnerable again and have become so self-sufficient and controlling that you have become isolated and cannot connect with others in a meaningful way. You will want to work with the Navel Fire to stabilize and contain your fire. In both cases, working with the Root Bowl and Sacral Lotus are also helpful, depending on your underlying emotional patterns.

FOUR
Heart Star: Your Center

Related Chakras: Your heart, or fourth, chakra

Energies: Love, compassion, balance, peace, equanimity, generosity, connectedness, humor, joy

Use For: Unworthiness, loneliness, hypercriticalness, coldness, jealousy, emotional upheaval, overwhelm, stress, tension, stinginess, greed, heaviness, humorlessness, joylessness

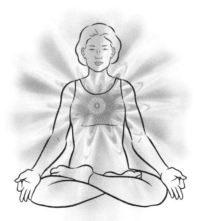

If you are new to the chakras, you may be thrown by the green color of the light in the Heart Star. In the West, we depict Valentine's hearts as pink or red and think of green as the color of envy. But the green of the Heart Star is the green of new spring leaves and healthy foliage. Think of the oxygen created by the plants around us, which is so intrinsic to our survival. In this way green represents pure air, and through that it represents breathing—the fundamental cycle of our body. The heart chakra is linked to both this and the fundamental energy of our psyche and spirit—love. To receive and give love is as essential to us as oxygen, and our heart chakra is the primary center through which this occurs.

The heart chakra also represents the center of our being. In the seven-chakra system, the heart chakra is right in the middle, with three chakras below it and three above. The heart chakra therefore represents balance—the balance between the energies of our lower and upper chakras, our inner and outer selves, our own needs and the needs of others, and giving and receiving. It represents our balance in our relationships with others. The heart chakra is our relational center.

We talk about love in relation to the people in our lives in two different ways. On the one hand, we speak of it as an emotion that comes and goes, like feeling happy or sad. But on the other hand, we talk about "loved ones," to refer to a core group of people in our lives all of the time, even in a moment when we aren't feeling the emotion of love toward them. The emotion of love may come and go, depending on what is going on between us and one of these core people, but if we are asked in a broader sense, "Do you love them?" we still say yes.

We also talk about love in a much broader sense, as a state of being. In a spiritual sense, when we talk about living from a place of love or acting with love in the world, we don't mean love in relation to a specific person. We are talking then of love as a state, as a force that we can connect with, and that can come through us, guiding the way we live. In virtually every religious tradition, love is considered a divine force, and a reflection of divine power.

So what is it that ties these different forms of love together? Connection and commonality. All the different forms of love that we experience spring from a deep sense of connection and commonality. We feel some part of ourselves in another being or beings. A spark in us is connected to a spark in them. This is true whether we are talking about romantic love, parental love, love of our friends, or a broader love of humanity, animals, or spirit. Opening ourselves to feeling this connection, to sensing this spark, is what the Heart Star is all about.

All of these forms of love are expressions of the heart chakra, and a lot of our work on the heart chakra is about separating out these kinds of love from attachment. Attachments are based on need and what we want from others. We may want validation, the feeling of worthiness, security, flattery—what-ever it is, when our relationship with someone is based on attachment, how we feel about them in any given moment is dependent upon whether or not we are getting what we want or think we need from them. Most relationships are a combination of love and attachment, so when we work with the Heart Star, we are seeking to clarify this for ourselves and empower our own ability to receive and give love that is based on connection, not attachment.

Empathy and compassion—our ability to feel others' pain, and our feeling of wanting to help them relieve it—are also linked to the heart chakra. Again, it is about connection and seeing past what we need from another person so that we can see and feel what they need from us. This act is another way we open our hearts. Many people—women in particular—are too open in this way, prone to putting others' needs above our own. This may be because we have not owned our own power enough to know what we need, because we are conditioned to believe that our own needs don't matter, or because we believe on some level that our worth derives from meeting others' needs. If this is you, working with the Heart Star is as much about learning to receive as it is about learning to give.

The heart chakra is not only about love and compassion. It is also about balance and the related states of equanimity, inner peace, humor, and even silliness. When we balance the giving and receiving of love in our lives, when we balance our own needs against the needs of others, when we achieve a calm inner state of balance and well-being, we gain a vast perspective on life that allows us to laugh. We don't need to grip life so tightly, squeezing hard to make sure that all our needs are met. We can let go and see the humor in it all, enjoying ourselves. This too is part of the beautiful shifts that the Heart Star can help enable within you.

Rochelle was a counselor at a domestic violence shelter, and for twenty years her warmth, vibrancy, and seemingly limitless energy had been an anchor for the women and children in her care. But now she was struggling, feeling burnt out and resentful. She felt disconnected from her work, and with personal problems of her own, she had a harder time feeling compassion for those in her care. She felt guilty about this and thought maybe it was a sign she should leave her line of work and do something else.

Rochelle's adult son was struggling with addiction, which had placed a lot of emotional and monetary strain on her. It was clear she had a lot of hurt and pain from this. She also babysat often for her adult daughter's children, and although she loved her grandchildren, she wanted to cut back on this childcare but didn't want to disappoint her daughter. As it turned out, there were many people Rochelle offered her services to in one way or another and many she did not want to disappoint. Rochelle put everyone else's needs before her own and had done so for a long time. She had hit her breaking point … there was nothing left to give.

I guided Rochelle through the Heart Star with special emphasis on the receiving portion of it. I asked her to visualize different people in her life and to imagine they were giving her light and love, which she received into her heart. Rochelle found great solace in her Christian faith, so she also visualized receiving this light from Christ. Finally she imagined emanating this light outward, fueled by an infinite source within her. Rochelle realized she had a lot of difficulty with receiving light and felt it was due to deep-seated patterns of unworthiness within her, leftover from a difficult childhood. She had spent her whole life trying to "make up" for these feelings, giving and giving, trying to be so "good" that eventually she would feel "good enough."

Rochelle worked with the Heart Star on her own for several weeks, focusing on receiving and a feeling of an unlimited source of light and love flowing to her and through her. After this time, we added in Second Skin work (an Empowerment later in this book), strengthening her boundaries and the ability to enforce them with others. Rochelle began to use both Empowerments throughout her day to enforce her boundaries and connect to the infinite source of heart light within her.

Rochelle began to feel connected to her work again, and to both self-compassion and her natural compassion for others. She realized she still cared about her work, but needed to carve out more time for herself, and create the space in her life to heal from her own pain, and to connect with family, friends, and healthy routines that kept her going. As she did so, she experienced a resurgence of both energy and inspiration.

Rochelle was experiencing a form of "compassion fatigue," a term used in therapeutic and medical communities to describe when individuals in healing and caretaker roles burn out from the constant barrage of need they face. Many women experience this fatigue to some degree, even those not in healing or caretaking fields because of the still disproportional role we play in childcare, elder care, and community support. Like Rochelle, many of us are also caught up in perfectionism or "good girl" syndromes, wherein we constantly try to make up for our own internal feeling of lack by being of service to others, seeking the validation through service that we are in fact good and worthy. Rochelle was a deeply compassionate person but was extending herself too far due to these patterns.

To be able to give, we must also be able to receive. We need to ensure we have the support we need and engage in the self-care required for us to have the heart energy to truly connect with others and offer our care as a true expression of love. Like flight attendants tell us on airplanes, we need to put our own oxygen masks on first before we can assist anyone else. Learning to receive and learning self-care are often the most important work we can do with the Heart Star.

When You Have Felt This Before

The heart chakra is an energy center that many people feel very physically from the start. To discover whether or not you do, think of a being you love in a very uncomplicated way—I often recommend a pet, a child, or a grandparent in your life. You can certainly think of your spouse, lover, parent, or friend, but our relationships with these people are often complex, which can make it harder to tap into your heart chakra energies immediately. You are really looking for a being for whom you feel an immediate sense of affection.

Imagine this being in front of you and cultivate the feeling of affection that rises up within you. Often it is literally a feeling of wanting to pull this being to your chest—your heart center—for a hug. Do you feel a warmth or tingle in the middle of your chest? If so, this is your heart chakra. It is not a problem if you don't feel it, but do imagine hugging this being to you—where is it you most want to connect in this hug? Often this is in the area of our heart chakra too. This feeling is definitely one you can use when seeking to activate the Heart Star.

Anytime you have felt love, compassion, or empathy for another being, you have felt the energy of your heart chakra regardless of whether or not you felt it physically. Think of times when you have witnessed the suffering of another being—animal or human—and felt that pain along with the deep desire to relieve it. Or think of any one of your loved ones and times in which you have felt held and supported by the feeling of being among them. These are all examples of heart chakra energy that you can draw upon.

And of course there's also the big LOVE—romantic love. When we are falling in love, it is intoxicating and even overwhelming. We may want to be with that person every moment of every day. At this stage of a relationship, there is lots of desire and attachment (and hormones!) mixed in with love, yet the drive to connect is still real and deep. It is also an example of heart chakra energy. If you can abstract from the feelings of desire and attachment and instead connect with this deep drive to connect, these memories of falling in love are also strong examples of heart chakra energy you can draw upon when working with the Heart Star.

Another way in which you may have already experienced the energy of the Heart Star in your life is through humor. I'm not talking about mean-spirited humor based on a feeling of superiority or ridicule of whoever is being made fun of, but joyful humor—true lightheartedness or even silliness. When you feel silly and lighthearted and are able to manifest or appreciate this kind of humor, there is a relaxation, a sense of letting go or releasing connected to the heart chakra. You suddenly see your predicament from a larger perspective and realize how ridiculous something is, how tightly you have been holding it. When you make fun of it or yourself, you are connecting with the lightness of your heart.

Feelings of peace, well-being, contentment, and tranquility are also emanations of your heart chakra. What in your life brings you these feelings, even for just a second? Watching the sunset? The sound of a bird in a tree? The feeling of calm when all your children are home for the evening? Anytime you feel or have felt these feelings of contentment, peace, well-being, and tranquility, you have also felt your heart chakra energies.

Generosity is also a heart chakra emanation. Think of a time in which you truly wanted to give, not out of a feeling of obligation or morality, but simply because you felt like sharing. Your gift may have been material—monetary or physical—but it also could be emotional—spending extra time with a child who craves your attention or helping an elderly relative in a time of need. When we practice true generosity, we don't feel like it is an imposition, or that there isn't enough time or money or whatever to go around. True generosity has a feeling of opening and expanding, rather than a feeling of loss. This opening and expanding happens in the heart.

Activation Steps

As always, settle into your space, prepare the guided audio file if you are using it, and any recall memories that are relevant from the last section. Gaze at the Heart Star image for a few minutes to familiarize yourself with it.

Step 1: Place both hands over your heart chakra—in the center of your chest at your breastbone, between your breasts. Alternatively, you can hold your hands in a prayer position with your thumbs touching the center of your breastbone. Breathe into the point where your palm or thumbs are touching your chest.

Step 2: During the visualization you may keep your hands in place, or put them down. In either case, begin to visualize a tiny green star where your hands were touching your chest. This star is made of light that is the vibrant green color of new spring leaves. This tiny, vibrant green star is three-dimensional, radiating light in every direction within your body.

Step 3: If you are working with memories of when you have felt heart energy before, bring them to mind now. Select one or two or cycle through each until the feelings of love, compassion, peace, balance, or lightheartedness arise as a tangible feeling for you. Imagine these feelings fuel your Heart Star.

Step 4: Next, imagine that rays of green light are flowing into your Heart Star from every direction—above you, below you, in front of you, behind you, and every direction in between. You can visualize individuals who care for you generating some of this light, and/or any spiritual force you believe in. Eventually, let images of these beings dissolve; just see the light itself pouring in from all around.

Step 5: Imagine that as this light pours into you, your Heart Star grows brighter and larger. Eventually, rays begin to emanate out from your Star to the rest of your body. Take some time to feel and experience these spring-like green rays of light emanating from your heart to every part of your body—your fingers, toes, head … everywhere.

Step 6: See the green light restoring balance and generating soothing energy everywhere it goes in your body. If you are experiencing a specific emotional pain in your life—grieving from a loss, a betrayal, or simply hurt feelings—you can also imagine this light flowing to the part of you that feels this.

Step 7: Eventually, see these green rays of light overflowing to emanate outside your body into the world. See these rays emanating out to animals, people, the land, or just emanating out into the world and universe in general. The center of your heart is your brilliant Heart Star, and there is no sense of a limit to what can come through you.

Step 8: Settle back down into the visual of your own Heart Star without the visual of either receiving or giving. Allow yourself to feel centered, balanced, and peaceful. When you feel ready, say each of the affirmations associated with this Empowerment 1-3 times, striving to feel each one as you do:

> I am accepting.
> I am loved.
> I am compassionate.

I am at peace.

I am balanced.

I am generous.

Step 9: Note how you are feeling, and take your snapshot memory. Dissolve the visual but sit in the feeling of the Heart Star for a while longer. Open your eyes when you feel ready.

With the Heart Star, it's particularly helpful to highlight its three-dimensionality. Really try to imagine and feel that the rays of light are spreading above you, below you, in front of you, behind you, and radiating out all the way around you like a sphere. Your Heart Star is about your relationship with the world, and visualizing it in this way will enable you to tap into a deep psychological sense of relating to all aspects of the world and all beings sharing it with you.

When You Are Blocked

Ironically, one of the main ways a heart chakra block can manifest is as a fixation on finding love. Women in particular often project onto our idea of a soulmate every quality we feel will make us complete. The longing for relationship is really a longing to feel whole. However, that wholeness can never come from someone else, and if your longing overwhelms everything else in your life, it may signal feelings of lack or the emotional wounds of shame or unworthiness.

Of course I believe in romantic love and encourage it! The reality, however, is that many relationships are mired in attachment and codependency, with both partners stuck in a constant cycle of fulfilling and falling short of each other's expectations. It may sound cliché, but to truly love another, you must first love yourself—and your partner must love themselves too. For women in particular, opening the heart chakra is first about learning to love yourself, care for yourself, and allow support in—allow yourself to truly receive love. The work of the Heart Star is learning to both receive and give love. It is often the case for women that the initial work is on learning to receive.

If your ability to receive is blocked, it may manifest in a few different ways. You may be very guarded, sharing little with others, perhaps appearing cold or in some cases shy. You may be isolated or lonely, or so dedicated to doing everything yourself that you will allow no one to help you or see when you are struggling or hurting. Or a receiving block may manifest entirely differently—maybe you constantly seek assurance that you are loved and supported, even to the point of creating drama to trigger a comforting response from those around you … but it never feels like enough. No matter how much others try to give you, you never feel reassured—you can't believe they care and won't really let it in.

Jealousy is often a reflection of this type of heart block. If we feel jealous in a romantic relationship in which we have no rational reason to mistrust our partner, it often means we just cannot believe the person actually loves us (it's of course a different matter if we are involved with someone who betrays us or gives us reason to mistrust them). Whatever they may say or do, we cannot accept this is possible—we cannot really believe in our own lovability. This lack of belief in your own lovability might also reflect in the kinds of people you end up in relationships with—perhaps you settle for being treated with indifference, mistreatment, or even abuse.

If we feel jealous of other people in our lives—for example a friend's accomplishments or traits—we are struck in another kind of heart block: comparison. When we don't feel whole in our ourselves, when we feel we are lacking in some way, we are constantly comparing ourselves to others and coming up short. We may feel jealous of what we perceive they have that we don't.

This kind of jealousy is often linked with patterns of comparison and judgment. By "comparison" I don't mean a healthy competitive nature in which you sometimes measure accomplishment against another to spur yourself on; there is a place for that. If you are mired in constant comparison or are constantly internally judging others or yourself (and they usually go together), however, there is a feeling of lack in the heart. Comparison of this nature puts you on an emotional roller coaster: when you compare yourself to another or judge another and feel "better," the internal feeling of lack or unworthiness is temporarily assuaged, but then the next day (or moment), you may come up short in the comparison game and feel terrible about yourself.

This is similar to the pattern of creating crisis or drama in order to trigger being comforted or feeling loved by someone in your life; you may temporarily feel better, but ultimately it never feels like enough. These strategies we engage in to feel worthy or loved are really only bandages on our heart. Real healing and wholeness require discovering the source of love within us by loving ourselves. The heart chakra is our relational center, so our tendency is to reach outside ourselves first, but actually the opposite is needed—go inward, receive inward, and *then* extend outward with your heart energy.

It follows that if we feel we aren't enough, or don't have enough, we might have difficulty being truly generous, so stinginess is another reflection of blocks in the heart chakra. This might be stinginess with money or material goods, or it might be stinginess with compliments, affection, or displays of love. Of course, with all the games we play to obtain the feeling of being loved, you might also give and give in an attempt to feel "good enough," or to receive back gratitude or even dependency from others. With our hearts, the truth is always about the *intention* behind what we do. Seeing the truth requires a great deal of insight and honesty. Working with our hearts makes us feel very vulnerable, because we are looking at our deepest shadows. Self-protecting to avoid vulnerability is often involved.

If you do give too much without tending to yourself, you can end up fatigued or resentful or both. The heart chakra is about achieving balance, including between care for yourself and for others. Imbalance may reflect as a swinging in your overall energy level (which might also involve the root chakra) or it may be a swinging of emotions (in which case it often involves the sacral chakra). The most common form of heart chakra imbalance is a swinging between feeling good and bad about yourself—superior and inferior, arrogance and self-hatred. If you tend toward the arrogant side, you may then lash out at others; basically, you may be mean. Meanness is the harshest form of self-protection. If you tend toward self-hatred, then you may be at risk for serious self-harm.

Heart chakra blocks also often result in a lack of a sense of humor or a tendency toward mean humor as opposed to lightheartedness. If you can't laugh at silliness, be silly, or allow yourself joyful and fun humor—including poking gently at yourself in a harmless way—this can also be a sign of heart issues. Or if you are always serious, locked into a cerebral way of approaching the world with no openness to flow or spontaneity, working with the Heart Star may be in order.

When we are locked in any of these cycles, we are stressed, and stress itself is also a heart chakra block. It's not a coincidence that stress affects our physical heart too, in the form of high blood pressure, hypertension, and other heart issues linked to stress. We've already talked about stress in the context of other chakras, as stress is often a multichakra issue, whether caused by never feeling safe (linked to the root), feeling of a lack of control (rigidity in the sacral or power issues in the navel), and so on. And the particular stressed out feeling of being *overwhelmed* usually has a heart component.

When we feel overwhelmed, we do not have the internal balance to handle what's coming our way, or we don't *believe* we do, anyway. The balance needed for that is seated in the heart chakra. The Heart Star is not just about the rays coming inward and going outward, it's also about the center point. When we are centered there, we have equanimity—we are the calm spot in the eye of the storm. Whatever is raging around us, we can see it clearly and choose our response.

Using the Heart Star

As you can see, the heart chakra really is central to so many aspects of our being. And because it is our relational center, the core from which we relate to other people in our lives, it is one we can benefit from touching base with frequently. I personally flash upon my Heart Star many times a day, more than any other Chakra Empowerment. Here are examples of when you might activate the Heart Star in your day—through all the activation steps or just quickly through a visual flash on your snapshot memory.

- When feeling overwhelmed by thoughts of all you need to do or accomplish. You may also want to use the Root Bowl to help stabilize your energy body and quell feelings of anxiety or panic.

- Similarly, activate the Heart Star whenever you are feeling tense or stressed. Again, the Root Bowl may also be helpful if your core emotion is fear, but the Heart Star will connect you with equanimity and inner calm, from which you can better address what is going on.

- Just after an encounter that has triggered anger, especially if it was with a loved one. The Heart Star will help you to calm down, eventually leading you to gain some perspective on the encounter and choose your response. You may need the Navel Fire first for focus.

- After an encounter that has left you feeling unworthy or jealous—any situation in which you find yourself comparing yourself unfavorably to another. This includes reading social media posts, like that frenemy's announcement of a promotion or a coworker's pictures of their amazing vacation. Center in your Heart Star to connect with your own inner sense of self-worth and to let go of comparison.

- When you catch yourself engaged in judgmental or hypercritical thought streams about yourself or others.

- When you are feeling lonely or excluded. Perhaps you have just heard of a party you weren't invited to, or overheard coworkers in a friendly exchange that you were not included in. Allow the Heart Star to help bring healing to this painful feeling.

- Just before spending time with a loved one(s)—the Heart Star can be especially helpful as a transition Empowerment, as you switch energetic gears between work and home.

- Just before a conversation with a loved one that you know may be difficult and you want to enter into with compassion.

- When you are feeling depleted and need to receive support and healing. Of course, you may need to reach out for help from actual people in your life depending on the issue, but touching base with your Heart Star can provide the first step. In some circumstances, it may be all you need.

- Anytime you are feeling humorless, joyless, cold, or out of touch with your kinder, compassionate side. In the busyness of our lives, it is easy to disconnect from our heart.

- Whenever your feelings are hurt. We are such sensitive creatures; many times a day we experience little bumps and bruises to our heart. Activate the Heart Star to connect to a deeper level, a level of your heart in which you are always whole and loved. Allow this level to heal and soothe the surface-level abrasions that involvement in the world creates.

You may want to work with the Heart Star daily for an extended time when you are working through long-standing patterns of feeling unworthy, hypercritical (of yourself or others), depleted, jealous, or overwhelmed. You may also want to work with it when you are emotionally hurting. Of course, as I have already mentioned many times, this chakra work isn't meant to replace therapy or counseling when you need it but is an excellent complementary tool for personal change and healing. In some cases, may be all you need.

Here are some more specific examples of when intensely working with the Heart Star in the longer term may be helpful:

- When you are working to create a sense of self-worth fueled from within, not based on others' perceptions of, or projections onto, you.
- When working to heal from deep emotional pain or trauma. Flooding your body with this healing, loving energy will help you through the most difficult phases of deep personal work.
- If you feel you are locked in patterns of judgment and criticalness toward yourself or others. This especially may become a pattern in marriages or long-term relationships; working with the Heart Star daily when you are working on healing a troubled relationship may be very helpful.
- If you are in a very stressful period of your life, interpersonally or regarding deadlines or pressure at work or other areas of your life. The Heart Star will empower inner balance and equanimity.
- When mourning the end of a relationship or grieving the passing of a loved one.
- When embarking upon, or engaged regularly in, service work with others.

At age thirty-four, Susan had never been in a relationship for more than a few months and was starting to panic, as she believed "time was running out." She mostly met men through an online dating site, which was something she found demoralizing but believed was her best option in the large city she lived in. She would frequently spend a lot of time speaking with someone over the phone first, only meeting in person if she felt there was a rapport. Usually she was disappointed when they met, believing that most of the men fell short of her expectations. In the rare cases where dating continued for a time, Susan was usually the one to call it off, always feeling that there was no long-term potential.

Susan wanted to work on changing what she called her "attraction field," as she thought the issue was that she was attracting the wrong kind of men. I suggested we work with the Heart Star to start, and then guided her through it. She found it very difficult to imagine receiving energy inward. She eventually relaxed and was able to feel it a bit, and then it triggered an avalanche of emotion. At first, she let loose a river of bitterness and anger at all the men she had dated, listing all of the things wrong with them, and all of the ways they had wronged her. After this settled, I asked her if she had grown to care for any of the men, and eventually she admitted that there was one, and that she felt very hurt by his eventual disinterest. I asked her to focus on the Heart Star every day for a week, especially on receiving, and to imagine some of the green light was going to the hurt she felt inside over rejection from the various men she had dated, especially this one.

After this, Susan reported a shift. She now felt that maybe the problem was her, that she couldn't receive positive energy, and so couldn't connect with the men she met. She listed all of the ways that she was terrible at dating and at relationships. She wanted to work on being better at both. I suggested we do the Heart Star again and focus this time on receiving and directing some of that light toward the part of her self-criticizing. As in our first session, this triggered a strong emotional reaction. Susan listed all of things she disliked about herself. I asked her to bring Heart Star light to this feeling, and she began to let go of this self-judgment. Susan began to laugh, saying, "I spent our first session criticizing every man I've ever dated, and now this one criticizing myself, didn't I?" With this realization, she began to see the pattern—the internal judge who was always operating in her mind, about herself and others, functioning as both self-protector and self-destroyer.

After this, Susan took a break from dating. She worked with the Heart Star to cultivate a true feeling of wholeness. She entered therapy for a time to work through contributing childhood issues. She engaged in more self-care in her life, including working out and eating healthier. She spent more time cultivating friendships, and tried to let go of the constant, disappointing search for the "right" man. She worked with the Heart Star throughout her day whenever she found herself judging herself or others, or whenever she started feeling stressed that she was not in a relationship.

As sometimes happens in these cases, a great partner was right in front of her. Susan had a neighbor she had known for years, and who had indicated some interest in her, but she had always dismissed him, saying he was not her type. As she got to know him better through their everyday interactions, she began to realize he was kind, intelligent, and funny. She realized she had written him off because he had not met the criteria on her internal "check-list" of the type of man she saw herself with. Their friendship blossomed into dating, and they are now married and have started a family.

It's often said that you'll find love as soon as you stop looking, and Susan's story is a classic example of this. In her case, the potential for love had been right in front of her for some time but she wasn't open to it—she was operating from a feeling of lack within her that caused her to search outside herself. From there, she would always find her partners or herself lacking. She also had set expectations for a partner based on a list of qualities she thought a potential partner had to have, which she eventually realized was oriented around traits she feared she didn't have herself. In addition, she had put pressure on herself to find someone quickly as she was worried about her biological clock and had bought into the idea that she was running out of time. Once Susan began to let go of all of this baggage and focus on self-love and self-care, everything shifted for her and she was open to love. In her case, she didn't even need to meet someone new—she just had to be ready and able to love herself.

Of course, what happened to Susan doesn't always happen; there are no guarantees in love. What's important is that when you develop self-love, you will be OK no matter what happens. Pairing off just for the sake of it—which women receive a lot of pressure to do—is never the answer. Anyone who has been through a difficult break up or divorce will tell you that the pain of a dysfunctional relationship is some of the harshest we can experience. You want to be grounded in self-love or working toward it when you are looking for or in a relationship. To be clear, no one is perfect—this work is not about waiting until you have "perfected" your self-love before seeking relationship … that can be another kind of trap. Relationships are a process of learning to love in and of themselves, and your ideal partner is someone willing to walk this path with you.

Women's Energetics: Pathways of Energy

So far, we have mostly looked at each chakra in isolation, although we have explored how you might use some Chakra Empowerments together. In reality, the chakras are a holistic system; the flow between them is as important as the individual energies. There are several ways our chakras are connected to each other we will work with later; connections between specific groups of chakras I call *pathways*. There are four main pathways:

- The upward pathway, moving energy from the root to the crown, associated with personal growth and spiritual realization.
- The downward pathway, moving energy from the crown to the root, associated with manifesting—turning ideas into reality.
- The masculine or yang pathway, connecting energies between the root (first), navel (third), throat (fifth), and crown (seventh) chakras. This is a pathway of emanating energies out into the world.
- The feminine or yin pathway, connecting energies between the sacral (second), heart (fourth), and third eye (sixth) chakras. This is the pathway of receiving energies from the world.

This last pathway is the reason I am bringing up pathways at all; in addition to being the center point of our entire seven-chakra system, the heart chakra is also the center point of the feminine energy pathway in our energy body. While we will work more formally with this pathway in the Feminine Pathway Empowerment chapter, understanding its connection to our sacral chakra is key. When we work on any one chakra in a pathway, we strengthen the entire pathway. And when one chakra is weak, the entire pathway is weakened.

While these pathways are all present in everyone, the feminine pathway is the central energy pathway in women's energy bodies, just as the sacral chakra is the ground zero of our energy body. This means the sacral, heart, and third eye chakras are especially important for us. They are also the most receptive and sensitive of the chakras in the chakra system. While all chakras have an emanating and receptive mode, the "default" setting on these chakras is receptive. For most women, this translates into a high level of energetic sensitivity throughout our entire energetic system.

We'll talk more about this energetic sensitivity later on, but I introduce it now to help provide some context for the role heart chakra work plays in most women's lives. We are often conditioned to define ourselves according to our relationships, and to place great emphasis on cultivating and maintaining relationships of all types—we experience our lives through a heavily relational lens. This makes us hyperattuned to how others react to us on a moment-by-moment basis. Social media has only exacerbated this tendency. Focus on others' reactions and responses to us—whether we are reading others' facial expressions for approval or waiting for likes on a post—is all experienced energetically through the relational center of our heart chakra. Our heart centers can easily become unmoored like pieces of driftwood in the surf, thrown about by the waves of others. The important work of the heart is to center our self-worth inward, rather than on this outward storm.

From an energetics perspective, the center of the Heart Star is this anchor point. When we are fully centered in this inner core, the ups and downs of relational shifts and reactions happen on the surface and do not determine how we feel about ourselves. It is like the calmness in the depths of the ocean, beneath the surface turmoil of the waves. We aren't pieces of driftwood being thrown around anymore. Whatever happens, we are anchored.

For women, this is the most important work we can do with our heart chakra. Anchoring it in this way stabilizes our feminine pathway and our entire chakra system. It helps us break the habit of defining ourselves and basing our self-worth on others' reactions to us. It is essential to breaking codependency and patterns of abusive relationships. And it's essential to finding a loving partner, if that's what we want, because then we aren't searching from a place of trying to fill a hole or a feeling of lack, but from an inner place of knowing who we are.

Sexual Trauma Healing: Relationships as Mirrors

For women sexual trauma survivors, the impact to the heart chakra is often a magnification of the patterns we've just discussed. The feelings of shame can create deep-seated feelings of unworthiness that result in an unmoored heart chakra, completely at the mercy of others. Mistrust is also a huge issue for obvious reasons, and it can deeply affect the kinds of relationships survivors are able to have.

Often our relationships are mirrors that reflect limiting self-beliefs, especially our romantic relationships. You may be drawn repeatedly to the same type of partner, wherein each reflects a particular emotional pattern. Some examples:

Someone who treats you poorly or is abusive
- Reflects feelings of unworthiness, replaying of childhood abusive dynamics.

A father figure
- Reflects need for paternal approval from either the mentoring/nurturing father you didn't have *or* the domineering father you did have.

Someone safe, i.e., platonic
- Reflects desire to avoid dealing with complicated feelings about your sexuality or desire.

Someone unavailable, married, or otherwise unattainable
- Similar to above, this is often a way of avoiding dealing with the difficult issues a truly intimate relationship might involve.

Someone who needs you
- Reflects need to not feel like the "weak" one, and/or to seek worth through the feeling of being needed.

Superficial relationships or none at all
   • Another way to "protect" yourself from intimacy.

Perhaps you see a combination of these at work, or some other pattern. Think about what parts of you are reflected in the types of relationships you have had or are having. These patterns do not necessarily invalidate your relationships (except in the case of abuse); they simply show you where you are working on your heart and may help you clarify what you are working to heal/release, and what you would like to empower/affirm.

Also consider your other types of relationships—family and friendships. Female friendships are often a big heart "reflector," particularly for women who are abuse and trauma survivors. Our feminine connection to each other is often disrupted along with our feminine power. Healing this is an equally important part of this work.

For all women, looking at our relationships from the perspective of the self-beliefs they reflect is important heart chakra work. But for sexual trauma survivors in particular, working to heal underlying pain and feelings of unworthiness by working with the Heart Star will help you strengthen your feminine chakra pathway and your entire energy body. On an emotional level, it will provide you a foundation for redefining how you relate to others and the world.

FIVE
Throat Matrix: Your Voice

Related Chakras: Your throat, or fifth, chakra

Energies: Communication, self-expression, listening, authenticity, clarity, honesty, integrity

Use For: Shyness, people-pleasing, difficulty speaking, compulsive speaking, dishonesty, confusion, inauthenticity, isolation, or to empower expression and communication of any type

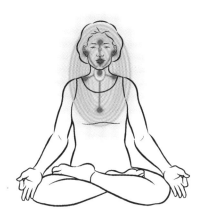

The throat chakra may be the most misunderstood of the chakras. It is linked to communication, and, accordingly, speech through the vocal cords in our throat. However, we can gain a deeper understanding of the throat chakra by considering the true nature of communication. Is it simply saying words, or is it getting our point across? I think we'd all agree it's the latter; after all, vocalizing a thought doesn't automatically mean we are understood. For effective communication, we not only need the ability to vocalize, we need the ability to *connect*. And connection requires listening and observing as much as it does speech. We must attune to how others react to our speech and adapt our words accordingly.

The throat chakra is linked to both sides of interaction—speaking *and* listening. It is about receiving inward as much as it is about expressing outward. It is an energetic bridge between ourselves and others. It is also a bridge within us between our inner and outer selves. How does anyone know what we are feeling or thinking? How do we know what anyone else is feeling or thinking? Through communication. It might be through speech or other means—body language, facial expressions, writing, sign language, signals. All of these are throat chakra functions on an energetic level. All of them are also ways of connecting our internal self with the external world.

What we actually communicate in any given moment—our external self—may be in or out of alignment with how we are truly feeling. We may speak our truth regularly, or we may hide it. We might calibrate our speech according to the reaction we want from others, prone to people-pleasing or grandstanding. We can use our speech to connect with people or deceive them—as a bridge or a wall. In this sense our throat chakra has a much deeper function—it is the compass of our authenticity and integrity.

The throat chakra serves as a bridge within our overall energy body as well. While the heart chakra is the center point in our seven-chakra system, the throat chakra is the gateway between our earthly and spiritual chakras. Our third eye and crown chakras are esoteric and spiritual in nature, much less linked to the energies of the material and human world than our root through heart chakras. In this sense our throat chakra is the gateway between our everyday energies, and our higher intuitive and spiritual abilities. If our lower and upper chakras are not linked through our throat, we may feel as if our lives are not in alignment with our "real" self.

In this age of social media, we emphasize speech and expression, but often devalue authenticity and connection. Receiving likes and hearts on our social media posts generates an endorphin rush and can easily lead us down a path of speaking and expressing solely to elicit this response, rather than as a true means of communication. When this happens, a disconnect occurs between our inner and outer selves, a disruption in our throat chakra. We have a lot of this kind of noise in our lives these days, and it is actually one of the primary throat chakra obstructive forces. Of course, social media and media in general offer us the unprecedented opportunity to find and connect with others. Navigating this effectively is part of throat chakra work.

The throat chakra has a much more ethereal side to it too. It is not only about speech but about *sound* and vibration as sound. Sound is linked in spiritual traditions to primordial energy—the sound of the Sanskrit mantra *Om* or *Aum* is considered a direct expression of the source energy of the universe. Music is sound with a direct link to our emotions, bypassing our linguistic mind. Music, mantras, chimes, gongs, and other forms of sound all function vibrationally, transporting us—shifting us energetically. We process these sound vibrations through our throat chakra.

The throat chakra empowers much more than speech. It bridges our inner and outer selves and is therefore linked to our sense of authenticity and alignment. It provides a gateway between our everyday and spiritual chakras and processes all sound vibration, including music and mantra. It is the center of a constantly functioning feedback loop in which we are both receiving and emanating sound and meaning. It is this entire loop and all of its forms that the Throat Matrix Empowerment is designed to clear and empower.

Karen had just turned fifty and was going through a divorce. She had difficulty at first articulating to me what she wanted to work on and answered questions in a very brief querying tone, as if she were checking in with me to see if her answers were okay. She mostly provided an overview of events without any sense of how she was feeling or her emotional state. She did share that she was attending a support group for new divorcées a friend had recommended, but so far she was uncomfortable with it and had never shared anything about herself with the group.

I decided to guide Karen through the Throat Matrix to see if we could open up her communications. After several minutes of activating the Throat Matrix, I asked her, "If you could say absolutely anything to your ex-husband right now, what would it be?" She angrily replied, "Well, that will never happen, because we only talk through our lawyers." She then immediately apologized for "snapping." I told her this was an imaginary exercise and to really imagine that if he was standing here right now, what would she say?

Once she started speaking, it was like a dam broke—a slight crack at first, a trickle getting through, and then a torrent. She expressed her sense of shock and betrayal at his sudden announcement that he was leaving; from her perspective, everything had been fine. She wanted to know why he was doing this and how he could inflict so much pain on her and their children. She laid into him for his selfishness and coldness and described her own humiliation at not being able to speak to him directly after so many years of marriage. When she was done, she immediately apologized to me for "burdening" me with her "outburst."

I talked to her about the bridge function of the throat chakra and how important it was for her to speak her true emotions in some setting—with me, friends, a therapist, or her support group. She shared how difficult this was for her to do, having grown up in a stoic household where emotional displays were considered indulgent or disobedient. She had spent her entire life holding her emotions in, rarely even arguing with her husband. She was adept at controlling her speech, feeling out what others did or did not want to hear and adapting accordingly. I asked her to do the Throat Matrix daily until our next session along with the Heart Star for healing and comfort.

In subsequent sessions and in her group therapy, Karen began to talk more about how she felt and realize how rarely she ever expressed what she really felt or thought. She realized that speech to her was about giving people what they wanted, and that she was especially angry about her divorce because despite sacrificing herself in this way, she was being left. She realized that in addition to her parents' stoicism growing up, she had also feared her father's fiery temper and quick mood changes. Although he had never been physically abusive, she had learned to adapt her words according to what

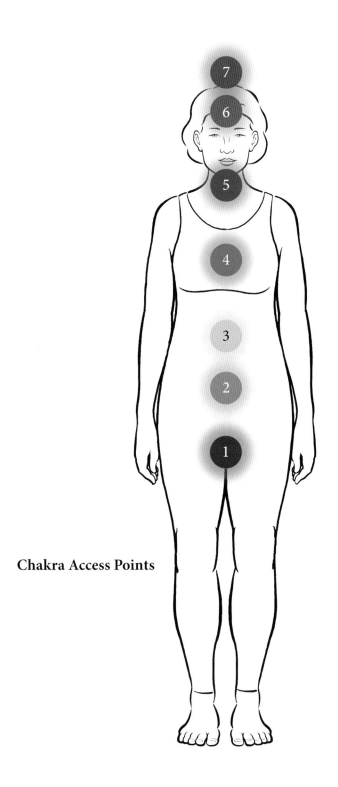

Chakra Access Points

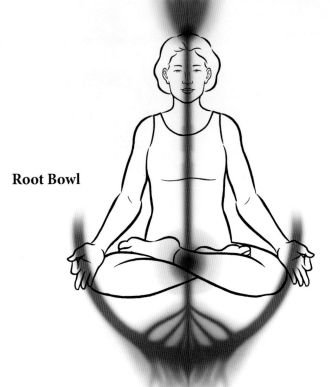

Root Bowl

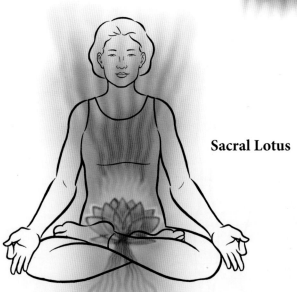

Sacral Lotus

Navel Fire

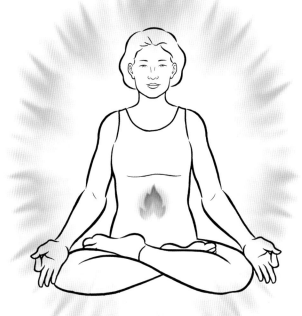

Heart Star

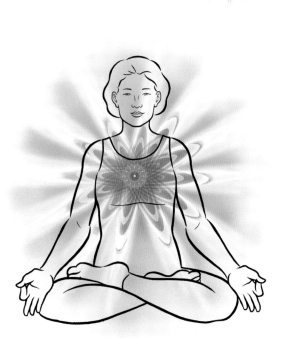

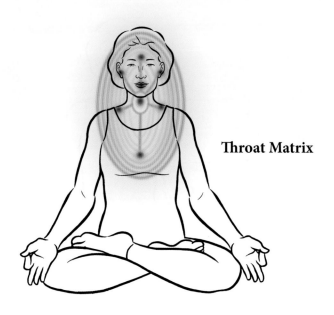

Throat Matrix

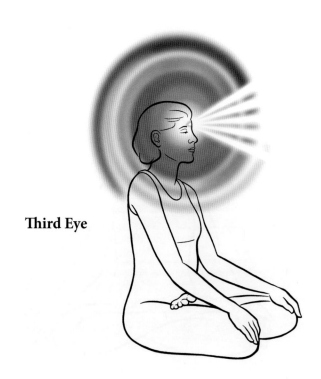

Third Eye

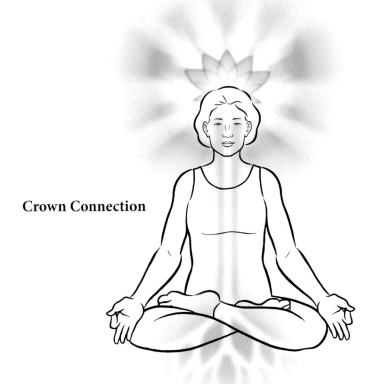

Crown Connection

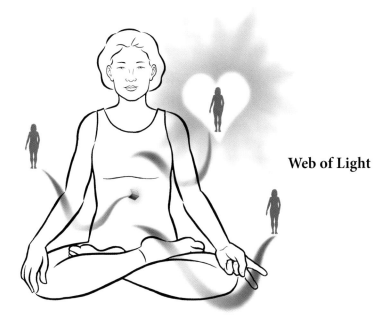

Web of Light

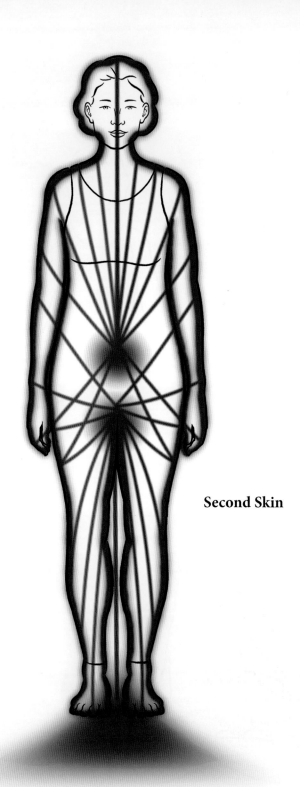

Second Skin

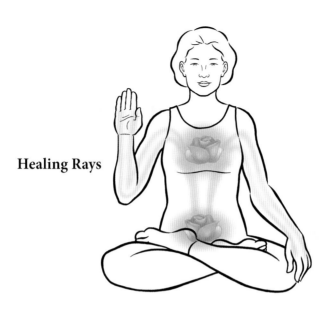

Healing Rays

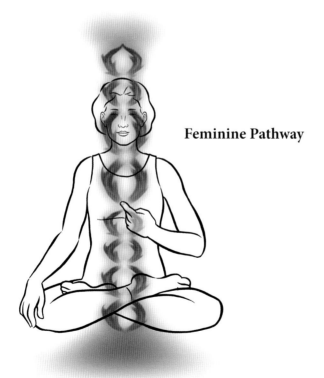

Feminine Pathway

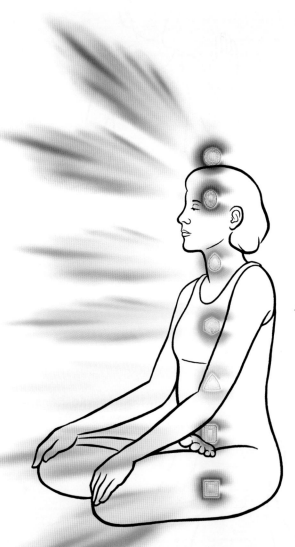

Rainbow
Abundance

might placate him or keep her under his radar. Her entire relationship with speech was about self-protection, not self-expression.

Karen continued to work with the Throat Matrix, as well as other Chakra Empowerments, particularly the Navel Fire, to empower her ability to speak her truth. She had honest conversations with her children and friends about what was going on and what she was feeling. With her teenaged children, she found that far from traumatizing them, as she had feared, her sharing opened up communication with them; they were encouraged to share their feelings with her too. With time, Karen moved through this difficult phase of her life and began to plan a new future.

Karen is a classic example of someone for whom speech (and communication in general) served as a wall rather than a bridge. When we are focused on saying what others want to hear rather than our truth, no one ever knows who we are and we end up feeling isolated. Of course, effective and compassionate communication isn't always about saying exactly how we feel when we feel it, but it is about connecting enough to how we and others feel so that we can make a skillful decision.

When You Have Felt This Before

If you are fortunate enough to have people in your life with whom you can truly share how you feel, those moments in which you have done so are prime examples of when you have felt your throat chakra energies before. You may also have felt these energies when you were *listening* in an open way or engaging in an open and honest exchange. When you are in a deep and thoughtful conversation with someone, truly hearing what they have to say, and feeling that they are hearing you back, the entire energetic loop represented by the Throat Matrix is open and clear.

Moments when you have spoken your truth when it was difficult, perhaps speaking truth to power, are also great examples of when you have felt your throat chakra energies in an empowered state. I don't mean angry outbursts; these usually have a lashing out quality because we are more focused on hurting another than speaking truth. Anytime you have felt as if you were saying something you really needed to say despite knowing that the person or people you were speaking to did not want to hear it is a memory you can draw upon.

If you are a writer or artist, and you use your medium as a form of self-expression, then you have also felt this aspect of the throat chakra. Think about the feeling you have when creative expression is flowing freely. Although other chakras are involved in the entire creativity cycle—the sacral for inspiration, the navel for execution, the third eye for imagination—the throat is linked to the actual expression, or communication, aspect.

If you sing, you have very directly experienced the energy of your throat chakra. You don't have to be a professional singer or performer—the shower counts! Try it if you can; focus on the feeling of the vibration in your throat and the flow of the sound through your throat and out your mouth. You could do this with mantras or chanting as well.

Listening to music, and especially being emotionally touched by it, is also an example of feeling throat chakra energies. Your emotional response to the music and the shift that takes place as you hear and process the sound, is conducted energetically through your throat chakra. Experiment with focusing on the vibration of the sound and the direct impact it has on you to connect with this aspect.

You can use memories of any of these kinds of moments to help you activate your throat chakra through the Throat Matrix. Although the great thing about the Throat Matrix is that you can also use sound right in the activation steps through chanting or humming or even singing to help you connect to this feeling.

Activation Steps

As always, settle into your space and body, prepare your memories and audio file (if you are using it), gaze at the Throat Matrix picture to familiarize yourself with it, then begin.

> *Step 1:* Center into your seated position, align your spine, and take a few deep belly breaths.
>
> *Step 2:* Place two fingers gently on your vocal cords, and do a light hum, mantra, or song note to locate the vibration there.

Step 3: Right beneath the spot where you feel this vibration most prominently, picture a luminous blue light. You can experiment with the exact color blue. I like a sky blue color because it evokes a sense of spaciousness and vastness, but you can visualize a brighter blue if you prefer. For two to three hums, chants, or notes, visualize this radiant sphere of blue light growing brighter under your fingertips, fueled by the sound vibration. Then stop creating sound and just picture the blue sphere in silence. You can drop your fingers from your throat at this point.

Step 4: Now visualize two additional dots of light at your ears and imagine a radiant line that connects the sphere at your throat and these two new ear lights. Focus for a moment on this visual of three lights, one at your throat and two at your ears, all connected.

Step 5: Add two more dots right at the base of your neck, where your neck transitions into your shoulder space. Visualize lines extending from your throat out to these connection points between your neck and your shoulders. Hold the visual of these five blue lights connected by lines.

Step 6: Add two final nodes of light, one at your forehead, and one down in your heart chakra. You now have the complete visual of a brilliant blue light in your throat, with six lines of blue light radiating out to points at your forehead, chest, each ear, and each side of your neck. You have a matrix of radiating light. See this entire matrix radiating out circles of light in addition to the flows of light between them.

Step 7: Sit with this visual for several minutes. If you like, you can return to creating sound and imagine the vibration is reverberating throughout this entire matrix of light.

Step 8: Speak the affirmations, focusing on feeling each statement:
I am honest.
I am clear with others.
I am authentic.
I am expressive.
I am receptive.
I speak my truth.

Step 9: When you feel ready, take your snapshot memory. Let the visualization dissolve and open your eyes.

Of course, if you are activating the Throat Matrix during your day in a setting in which you cannot make a sound, it's perfectly fine not to. But I encourage you to experiment with sound and vibration when you are in the initial stages of learning this Empowerment. Working with the Throat Matrix will strengthen your understanding of the affirmation process as well, because their power comes from our ability to connect with the feeling of what we are saying. Affirmations are not simply repetitions of empty words. Evoking a connection between the words we say and the associated feeling is itself a throat chakra function. So, make use of the Throat Matrix whenever you want to empower affirmations of any type.

When You Are Blocked

Similar to the navel chakra, most throat chakra blocks or weaknesses manifest in one of two opposing ways—either as *under*talking or *over*talking. Undertalking might reflect as shyness or passivity—a reticence to speak or interact at all. Or it might involve talking very quietly, in one-word answers, or in a very limited way that hinders any true connection with others. If you are an undertalker, you may actually fear speaking, or you may feel as if you would like to say more, would like to connect more with people, but simply can't, as if there were a wall in your being preventing you from doing so.

On the other hand, overtalkers talk a *lot* but do not say much or at least not much of significance. They may talk quickly and incessantly, leaving little room for anyone else to get a word in, and perhaps interrupting. Or they may spin, repeating themselves or going off on tangents that are hard to follow. They may compulsively overshare. Their verbal barrage becomes a wall; instead of connecting them with others, it pushes people away. And of course if they are always talking, it goes without saying that they are also not listening, so there is no sense of exchange.

Another manifestation of a throat chakra block or weakness is a habit of confusing, evasive, or dishonest speech. If you have trouble with any of these, you may genuinely want to speak clearly and honestly, but find yourself habitually unable to. Small lies, in particular, can become a form of self-protection or self-aggrandizement rooted in fear or a desire to gain approval from others. The psychological underpinnings of such behavior usually involve more chakras than simply the throat, but the manifestation of these speech tendencies always involve throat chakra dysfunctions.

A subtler form of throat chakra dysfunction is feeling that your inner and outer selves are not aligned. You may be very articulate and outwardly have no sign of communication problems but feel as if the person you present to the world has nothing to do with who you are inside. This is in fact one of the more common ways that sexual trauma or childhood abuse of any type may affect the throat chakra. If you grew up forced to keep secrets about what was happening in your household or had to hide part of your experience, a wall may have been created between your inner and outer selves. At some point, this wall becomes an actual energetic block of the gateway aspect of the throat chakra—the function it serves of connecting your inner and outer worlds.

Another throat chakra dysfunction is an inability (or refusal) to comprehend what others say. We may hear the words but not process what is being said. We might feel confused or simply block out certain truths that we do not wish to face. Linked to disassociation, this latter tendency also usually has ties to other chakra issues but is largely reflected in the throat chakra.

An inability to listen to or appreciate music or any sound can also be a kind of throat chakra dysfunction. Of course, not everyone has to love music or music of all types. But if you really cannot appreciate music at all, it may be a sign of a general block against sound vibration, and that can mean you are blocking out other levels of energetic sensitivity that may actually be useful or pleasurable for you. Because of its function as a vibrational sensor, our throat chakra is linked to our overall vibrational sensitivity.

Using the Throat Matrix

It is probably very clear to you which types of situations might call for activating the Throat Matrix: before any encounter in which your speech or communication is particularly important. Which aspect of your communication that you seek to empower may vary according to your specific challenge and intention. You might need to strengthen your ability to speak in a stressful situation, or strengthen the power and volume of your voice. You might need to empower your clarity or authenticity. Or if you are prone to nervous overtalking, you might instead need to strengthen the connection between your inner and outer self as well as your ability to speak meaningfully and purposefully from your heart.

For some of these situations, you may want to include other Chakra Empowerments. If so, activate the other Empowerment first and then activate the Throat Matrix, since your speech is an expression of another aspect of your being. For example, if you are nervous about giving a big speech, you might first activate the Root Bowl to ground and stabilize your energy body and quell your anxiety. Then you could activate the Throat Matrix to empower your speech. Remember that once you have spent some time familiarizing yourself with these Empowerments, you can use your snapshot memory taken in the final step of each activation series to activate them very quickly—just a simple flash upon each for a few seconds will be enough.

Here are some other examples of when you might activate the Throat Matrix, in some cases with ideas for how you might combine this Empowerment with others:

- A conversation where you need to assert yourself and ask for something that is difficult for you. In this case you might first want to activate the Navel Fire and then the Throat Matrix.
- When you need to relay difficult news, something someone may not want to hear. You may want to activate the Heart Star too if you are relaying news that will be painful to someone.
- When you are seeking to motivate or inspire others. In this case, you may want to combine it with the Sacral Lotus to generate the feelings of inspiration.

The Throat Matrix is not only about empowered speech, of course; it is also about truly hearing and comprehending what others say to us. Here are examples of when you may use it in that context:

- Before heading into a performance review at work or any situation in which you are receiving feedback.

- Before a needed but potentially difficult conversation with a loved one—perhaps discussing with an elderly parent that it may no longer be safe for them to drive or confronting a teenaged child with falling grades.
- Before attending a lecture or talk in which you know the material may be challenging for you to comprehend, but which you are very interested in absorbing.

You may also want to activate the Throat Matrix in situations where you want to increase your authenticity, self-expressiveness, or vibrational sensitivity:

- Before a dinner party at which you don't know anyone well but would like to connect on a more than superficial level.
- When writing or composing an artistic piece that is an expression of your feelings or inner state.
- While listening to a concert or musical piece you want to connect with on a deep level.

Of course you may also want to use the Throat Matrix regularly for a time if you feel you have throat chakra–related blocks. Here are some examples of why you might work with it in this way:

- You feel that you hide or shield your true self from others through either under- or overtalking.
- You have patterns of compulsive people-pleasing or dishonesty rooted in insecurity or fear. You may also want to work with the fear or anxiety itself through another Empowerment or other therapeutic modalities.
- You are in therapy, alone or couples, to heal long-standing issues, and feel a need to open up your ability to express yourself honestly to your therapist and/or partner.
- You are involved in a creative project in which you are bringing forth deep parts of yourself—for example, the writing of a memoir, or an autobiographical artistic piece.

Your issue with speech may not be inauthenticity, it may be clarity. You can also use the Throat Matrix to help you improve your ability to communicate effectively through the spoken or written word—perhaps while you are engaged in a speech or writing class. You might use it (as I do) when you are involved in a writing project—not necessarily a creative writing project; it could be an application essay, presentation for work, or important email or letter. If you are a composer, songwriter, or musician, working with the Throat Matrix when you are writing or performing frequently may also be helpful.

Maia was twenty-six and a prime example of an overtalker. It was difficult to break into her narrative to speak, and while she clearly needed someone to truly hear her, it hindered our ability to do any meaningful energy work. She told me that her primary goal for our work was to help gain some financial stability. Although she had certification as a masseuse, she had never been able to make ends meet through it and had ended up jumping from job to job in the service industry.

When we spoke, Maia would typically begin with a story of some situation or encounter at work or with a friend that had triggered her and then tangent off into situations from her childhood that she believed had contributed to her being triggered. While often insightful, everything stayed decidedly on an analytic level, and it was difficult for her to express how she felt or where she experienced a particular emotion or energy in her body. Often it was difficult to ask these questions without deliberately interrupting her.

I asked Maia to first begin working with the Root Bowl to ground and connect with her body. Although she could connect with the exercise as we did it together, once she began talking afterward her energy surged upward, into her throat and third eye chakras, creating a hyperactivity there that then expressed through her talking and self-analysis. I described for her what I was sensing and asked her to do the Root Bowl daily between sessions, and to practice staying grounded in her lower chakras as much as possible, without popping upward.

We worked with Maia's root chakra for several weeks, focused on releasing blocks from past experiences that had hindered her ability to connect with her root and to stay grounded in it. Although Maia became more aware of her tendency to disassociate from her root, she continued to use her excessive speech as a wall at times, slowing further work. We then shifted into working with the Throat Matrix.

It was while working with the Throat Matrix that Maia really began to open up. She mentioned having been sexually abused by a family friend when she was between the ages of five and eight years old. Although Maia had very clear memories of what had occurred, she had only ever told one person, her mother, when she was around seven years old. Her mother reacted very angrily and accused Maia of lying, so she never spoke of the abuse again. In fact, Maia insisted that this abuse was not an issue, that she had moved through it on her own. Nevertheless, I encouraged Maia to continue working with the Throat Matrix and to consider journaling about her abuse if she felt it would not be traumatizing to do so. I also suggested she seek out counseling specifically around her abuse. She was not interested in counseling at that time but agreed to use the Empowerments and attempt some journaling on her own.

Over the coming weeks, Maia became more and more open about her abuse; more importantly, she was able to express the emotions she felt around it. She was able to express how angry she felt at her mother for dismissing her and not protecting her, how betrayed and angry she felt toward her abuser, and how much shame she had internalized over what had occurred. She was able to pinpoint where she felt these emotions in her body so we could work with them in other ways. Above all, Maia's entire way of communicating shifted; she was now able to engage in exchange with periods of truly listening and responding as opposed to creating a verbal wall through over-talking.

Maia eventually did pursue other forms of counseling and healing in addition to our work. With time, she was able to transform her life. Although her mother had died several years before, she spoke to her sister about her childhood abuse, who believed her, as she had memories of her own that validated what Maia remembered. This sharing and validation in particular played a huge role in Maia's transformation. As she faced and healed from her abuse, her need to disassociate from her lower chakras diminished, and

Maia was better able to stay grounded. We also aided her ability to financially sustain herself, her original goal in our work together.

Maia's story demonstrates the crucial role that true sharing and communication plays in our healing and growth process. Many of the challenges Maia faced in her life were related to her inability to stay grounded and manifest utilizing her lower chakras. But it was opening the gateway of authenticity in her throat chakra that paved the way for her transformation. Maia had kept the secret of abuse inside for so long and habituated using speech as a wall between herself and others. Once this secret was released, she no longer needed this wall and could begin to integrate her emotions and energy holistically, stay grounded and centered in her root chakra, and truly communicate and connect with others.

Women's Energetics: True to Yourself

For women at this time in history who are working to change long-standing cultural and social forms of oppression, the most valuable energy work we can do is empowering our navel and throat chakras in order to own our power and voice. Speaking up for yourself and speaking truth to power—whether in a personal relationship, workplace, or social context—is how the work unfolds.

One of the biggest conditioned patterns that many women have to break through in terms of owning their voice is the habit of using speech as a means to please or placate others. As we talked about in the Navel Fire chapter, girls are still rewarded for niceness, and women are often expected to be the relationship balancers and caretakers in couples and groups. This conditioning can function on a very subtle level and be difficult to see, so I encourage you to look for it, even if you feel you are a woman who speaks her truth.

One way to do this is to spend a few days keeping a communications journal. Keep a small notebook with you, and as you go about your day, pause after social interactions, and ask yourself, "Did I feel responsible for that situation in some way? Did I choose what I was going to say in order to elicit a particular response? Was I trying to avoid a response I didn't want to deal with? Was I placating or pleasing someone I was speaking to or who was present?" If you are very honest with yourself, you will likely find that you are doing this much more than you realize.

Of course, to some extent there is no problem with this. Sometimes we speak to elicit the response we want to influence people, placate them, or get them to like us. There is no problem with this … *if* we are aware of it and it is not the only way we are in the world. What you are looking for are the ways you have become habituated to this, the ways in which this type of speech has become your unconscious operating system—the extent to which you are communicating as a form of self-protection or validation instead of as a means of self-expression and connection.

Rewriting this pattern usually involves understanding the psychology beneath it, and changing it may involve other chakras. Here are some of the most common emotional foundations for this pattern, along with the combinations of Chakra Empowerments you might use to support your work to change them:

> *Fear:* If you grew up in a home in which you did not feel safe, or in which you could be severely punished for saying something deemed unacceptable, you may have developed communication patterns to create safety as a survival strategy. Perhaps you smooth over conflicts by changing the subject or making jokes, or perhaps you focus on placating the individuals with the most volatile personalities. You instinctively feel out and seek to manage the room or at least everyone's response to you in order to feel safe. Combining Throat Matrix work with Root Bowl work is the best energetic support for shifting this pattern.

> *Unworthiness:* We all want to be liked, but when we feel solid in our self-worth, we do not need *everyone* to like us or be validated in every social situation. If we harbor deep feelings of unworthiness or shame, we crave validation from others, often in the form of being liked. We may modify ourselves and our speech according to who we are with in order to fit in or to elicit praise, laughter, or a feeling of belonging. We can easily lose any sense of who we really are, trapped in an endless game of adapting to what people want from us. Social media often magnifies this trend, as we crave likes for our

posts as a form of validation. Combining the Sacral Lotus with the Throat Matrix will support work on shifting this pattern.

Responsibility: Women often are the social and energetic anchors for any group, whether in a family unit, social group, or work team. We may feel as if we must play hostess at all times and that we are responsible for how others are feeling. If someone is unhappy or displeased, we take it personally and feel we must address it, even if the setting in which it is occurring is not something we have organized or arranged. Releasing this sense of responsibility is about reclaiming our boundaries; as such, working with the Navel Fire (and possibly the Second Skin, introduced later in this book) along with the Throat Matrix will support you in letting go of this tendency.

Sexual Trauma Healing: Liberation from Secrecy

All the patterns outlined above may be magnified by the experience of sexual abuse or assault. If you were abused in your home as a child, you may have adapted your speech and presentation of yourself to keep yourself safe or to compensate for feelings of shame or unworthiness. If you were assaulted later on in your development, the experience may have shattered your sense of safety or worth, resulting in similar patterns from that point forward.

But there is another wound to the throat chakra that is more specific to sexual abuse and assault survivors—the pain of secrecy and silence. If you are a childhood sexual abuse survivor, your abuse was likely a secret, and perhaps your abuser manipulated or threatened you to make sure it stayed that way. As in Maia's case, perhaps you told someone but were not believed, and kept the secret from that point forward. Perhaps you sensed others knew what was happening but there was an unspoken agreement never to speak of it. Whatever form it took, your voice was stifled and you were forced to keep this painful secret—one that for many survivors creates a wall between themselves and others that feels impossible to surmount.

The situation is often very similar for adult assault survivors. A victim may never tell anyone of her assault or tell and not be believed. As well, in situations in which a survivor shares what occurred and presses charges, the legal process can feel disempowering and stifling. Even if a survivor of either abuse or assault does share her experience with loved ones, the response is not always affirming. Some people may be uncomfortable hearing about it or only want to discuss it once and then tell the survivor to move on or "get over it." These dismissive responses create a new veil of silence and can trigger a lifelong struggle to decide who and who not to tell. Many survivors report agonizing over the decision of when to tell a new friend or romantic partner about their history out of fear of how the person will handle it. When not shared, it can feel like a barrier to intimacy … but when shared, the result can often be the same.

The constant struggle over what to share with whom and when is for the most part unique in our society to sexual trauma survivors. Cancer survivors, accident victims, or victims of other crimes rarely feel the same conflict. On an energetic level, the struggle takes a toll, reflecting as a block or wall in the gateway function of the throat chakra. This block may manifest in any of the patterns we've discussed—undertalking, overtalking, people-pleasing, and so on. Working on dissolving this wall is one of the most empowering healing processes you can undertake as a sexual trauma survivor.

Working with the Throat Matrix for a period of time can support you in this process. If you have undergone or are engaged in counseling, it may serve as a forum for you to truly share what happened to you. Journaling your full experience or sharing it anonymously on a website designed for such purposes can also be powerful ways of breaking through this veil of silence and secrecy. You don't have to shout your experience from the mountaintops to experience healing, but opening up communication in some way is crucial.

Allowing yourself to identify and express emotions related to your trauma, especially anger, is also often critical to opening up the bridge between your inner and outer selves. Anger is an important step in the healing process that shouldn't be bypassed. Because I work with the chakras, I attract a lot of spiritually minded sexual trauma survivors. I find that many are hyperfocused on forgiveness. They feel that they "should," as adults, be able to forgive their abuser or assaulter. They say, "I know he/she was acting from his/her own damage." That may be true, but I've found that if the stage of anger is bypassed, it often leaves subtle blocks of self-blame and shame that are never surfaced and released. Allowing yourself to truly express anger—at your abuser, your assaulter, and anyone who failed to believe or protect you—is an important step in the healing process.

You can do the release of anger as a visualization exercise, perhaps supported by a counselor, healer, or friend, in which you visualize you are speaking to the person, or you can write it as a letter. It does not matter if you are ever able (or ever want) to actually communicate your anger to the person. The important thing is that you open the dam and let the anger out; in doing so, you place the blame for what happened squarely where it belongs—with your abuser or assaulter, *not* yourself. Perhaps in time, focusing on forgiveness will feel appropriate for you … or perhaps not. Personally, I don't think it's helpful to push forgiveness or expect it or hold it as necessary to move forward with life in a healthy and whole way. What's much more important is your relationship with yourself.

SIX

Third Eye: Your Second Sight

Related Chakras: Your sixth chakra, or third eye

Energies: Intuition, imagination, insight, wisdom, clear seeing, envisioning, potentialities, stillness, timelessness, boundarylessness

Use For: Confusion, mental fuzziness or fog, indecisiveness, lack of clarity, problem-solving, mental ruts, lack of ideas, or to empower insight, intuition, or imagination

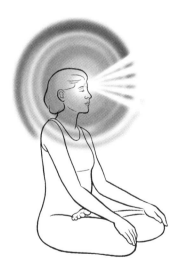

The sixth chakra is referred to as the third eye because it is linked to a subtler level of sight, a level of perception beyond our physical senses. We usually call this intuition, but a more accurate term may be "energy attention."

To understand what I mean, stop reading this book for a moment, and spend one minute focusing on every sound you can possibly hear in your current environment. You will discover there are all sorts of sounds around you that you had not been aware of—birds singing, the heater blowing, cars driving by, the light buzzing. These were all there before you noticed them, and your ears were receiving their sound vibrations—the sensory input. However, your mind screened them out—you did not *perceive* them—because your attention was on this book.

The interplay between senses, perceptions, and attention is mirrored in the relationship between our energy body, third eye, and intuition. Our energy body receives energy input from all around us, just as our physical senses receive sensory input … but we pay attention to very little of it. Our attention is usually elsewhere unless we deliberately train in developing our intuitive abilities, as most of us are never aware of how these energies affect us. But if we learn to pay attention to them and open our third eye, we can perceive things from this energetic data. This is how our third eye directs our energy attention.

The third eye is about abstract mental functions as well, particularly imagination and insight. These three "i" words—intuition, imagination, and insight—are the primary powers of our third eye. "Ideas" is another good third eye "i" word, because the third eye's energy fuels our ability to generate ideas. When our third eye is blocked or weak, we have little to no imagination, difficulty brainstorming new ideas, no intuitive guidance in our lives (relying entirely on rational thought) and have little self-awareness because we do not have the insight to bring this forth.

In today's world, most of us receive little support for developing our third eye. Growing up is often presented as a process of shutting down the natural, freewheeling imagination, intuition, and insight of our childhood. We are encouraged to "get serious," "make plans," and "face reality." The result is a lack of support for our third eye, even though making use of it could absolutely help us get serious, make plans, and face reality in an effective and fulfilling way! If you were an especially intuitive young child prone to visions or energetically sensitive, you probably received messages to shut these abilities down.

However, if you experienced trauma in your childhood, you may also have gone the other direction, developing patterns of disassociation that result in you living *too much* through your third eye without a connection to your lower chakras and their functions. This kind of disassociation involves disengaging from our lower chakras and living in our upper chakras, particular our third eye. We can become disengaged from communal reality, connection to others, our own emotions, and even physical sensations, to instead live in a realm entirely created through our imagination. Or we can become enthralled by "astral," dreamlike worlds available to us through our third eye. We may become convinced that we are receiving spiritual messages and signs in this way, but eventually they become so self-referential that we are no longer grounded in our bodies.

Working with the Third Eye Empowerment requires staying grounded and real. I've designed the activation steps for this Empowerment specifically to help you do this, as well as to help you maintain a healthy connection between your lower and upper chakras. This Empowerment does not open all of the functions of the third eye; we won't work with astral travel, for example, nor is it meant to serve as a full-scale method for developing your intuitive abilities. As with all the Empowerments in this book, the focus is on how you can use your third eye in your daily life and work with it for emotional healing and empowerment.

Natalie had been a high achiever her entire life, first as a student and athlete, and then initially in her job as a software engineer. But as she progressed in her career, she had hit a wall. After landing a prestigious job with a prominent technology company straight out of college, she found she had stalled after the success of her first few years. Through feedback, she had come to realize she had no vision. She was good at executing someone else's ideas but had few of her own. This tendency extended into her personal goals as well—she knew she wanted something more from her life but could not really imagine what.

Natalie was extremely intelligent and book-smart. We began working with the Sacral Lotus to help counterbalance her cerebral nature and connect to some new energy of inspiration and passion. However, she found it difficult to visualize. She was very concerned with creating the visual exactly right, trying to form it like a painting in her mind. She also had difficulty cultivating feelings associated with the affirmations. The entire activation process frustrated her.

I asked Natalie if she ever daydreamed: Did she ever replay a conversation from the past going differently in her head? Did she ever find herself fantasizing about a future event or encounter she would like to have? This she could relate to—she recounted daydreaming about an upcoming vacation she was looking forward to, imagining herself on a beach with a drink in her hand. We walked through the steps of activating the Third Eye Empowerment after which I asked her to describe her fantasy of this vacation in detail and flesh it out even more if she could. This went great, and Natalie was encouraged to realize that of course she did use her imagination all the time in this way. I asked her to activate her third eye daily between sessions, and to spend some time imagining this vacation she was looking forward to in detail for a few minutes afterward.

True to her high-achieving nature, Natalie was very diligent about this assignment and recounted all of her imaginings at the start of our next session. But she also had realized how guilty she felt using her imagination, like she was wasting her time. She realized that while growing up, she had been discouraged from using her imagination or intuition. At one point she had an imaginary friend—very common for young children—but when she told her mother about it, her mother told her to "stop making up that nonsense." At another point, she remembered having had a dream of an event that later came true. When she told her mother about this, she got an even angrier response. Natalie's parents had high academic expectations for their kids, so with time she squashed down her third eye tendencies and learned to direct her mind only to study.

We worked with Natalie's feelings of guilt at using these parts of herself as well as the feeling she had internalized that her intuition and imagination were not responsible or "safe." Our work involved activating both her Root Bowl and Sacral Lotus, which she was able to do with time in addition to working more with the third eye. Natalie began to connect with this part of herself again and eventually left her job to join a startup firm where she was a valuable part of the R&D team, including generating many new ideas. Over the long term, these shifts also led Natalie to explore spirituality, something that opened up even more dimensions of herself.

Natalie's experience growing up is very common, and of course her parents were well-intentioned in terms of wanting their children to succeed in the world. But it had caused Natalie to disengage from her third eye functions and to feel guilty whenever she did utilize them. As a result, she couldn't envision new possibilities in any other context, either. Opening our third eye isn't about becoming a professional psychic or artist—for most of us it is more about opening to a sense of possibility and potential for our lives. All change starts with vision of some type—that is what a goal is—and our third eye enables this kind of vision.

When You Have Felt This Before

Natalie's story highlights one of the most common ways you have most likely felt third eye energy before: through daydreaming. Although daydreaming and fantasizing can become dissociative or dysfunctional if we engage in them too much, they are a very important part of our visioning process in healthy moderation. By visioning, I mean the way we explore potentials for our future. Whether it's daydreaming about how you're finally going to quit a job you dislike, a trip you are looking forward to, the romantic partner you hope to meet, or that business you are going to start, daydreaming is part of the way you acknowledge your desires for your future.

Daydreaming is a form of imaginative thinking, and imagination is another key third eye function. As we've discussed, sacral chakra energy provides the boundary-breaking and inspiration energy for our imagination, but the third eye provides the form or content—what we actually imagine. So, if you innovate or create from a place of pure imagination within yourself, think about how it feels when you are doing so. You can tap into the memory of this feeling, too, to help activate the Third Eye Empowerment.

Another way you have already experienced your third eye energy is through your intuition. Everyone experiences intuition. A basic example of it is sensing someone is not quite sincere, lying, or that they are feeling differently than whatever they are presenting to you. For example, imagine you run into a coworker outside of work and chat for a while about how you both are doing. He tells you everything is fine, he is smiling and friendly, but you sense under the surface something is not right. Later you hear he is getting divorced or is going through some other difficult life experience. In retrospect it's clear to you that your insight was correct.

What did you sense? Body language? A difference in his tone? Rigidity? We pick up on all sorts of things that we aren't consciously aware of. From an energy perspective, you likely also experienced the energy of his underlying emotions—the energy of sadness or anger emanating off of him. Your energy attention may not have been on this feeling explicitly, but your third eye processed it.

To pinpoint the energy of your third eye as it functions in this way, draw upon a memory of a similar situation or any time you feel you had a flash of intuition. Other common examples are thinking of someone right before you get a call or text from them, or "knowing" you are going to find a parking spot around the next corner. The content of your memory does not matter, but you do want to work with a situation in which your intuition was later proved correct. Tune into this memory, pinpoint the moment the intuitive thought flashed into your mind, and then try to identify for yourself the feeling in your mind and body as it happened. With time, you will sense that these kinds of thoughts have a different feeling to them and that your mind and body feel differently when you are having them as opposed to other kinds of thoughts.

Accurate intuition goes hand in hand with another third eye function: insight. Without insight, we can easily think we are having an intuitive thought, when in fact our "intuition" is based in fear or past conditioning. For example, if you have experienced betrayal or dishonesty frequently in your life, you will likely be predisposed to thinking people are lying to you—and you may very well think these thoughts are intuitions. But if you have the insight to recognize this pattern when it arises, you can sort through what is fear and what is intuition. This insight function of our third eye is like our internal BS sensor. When our third eye is open and clear, it serves as an inner compass, always pointing to our true north and keeping us on track.

There is one final form of third eye energy you may have experienced in its spiritual expression. The third eye is closely linked to meditation and meditative states of deep stillness, timelessness, and boundarylessness. You might have experienced these in formal meditation or prayer, or spontaneously while in nature, a yoga practice, or even during your regular day while in a phase of your life that forced you to dig deep. If so, draw upon the memory of these experiences as well when you activate the Third Eye Empowerment.

Activation Steps

Prepare as usual: queue up the audio file if you are using it, prepare your space and memory list, and gaze at the Empowerment image.

Step 1: Sit with a straight back and place one hand over your navel chakra. Breathe deeply into your hand, experiencing the rise and fall of your belly under your hand as you do so. Take at least five breaths in this way. We will end in the same way—this is important for keeping you grounded in your body as you work with your third eye chakra.

Step 2: With your index finger, press firmly into your third eye focal point, the midpoint just above your brow line. Press and release several times, and each time you release, imagine you are relaxing more into the energy of this part of your body. This physical connection to your third eye focal point is another useful method for staying grounded in your body as you work with your third eye.

Step 3: Drop your hand down; right where your finger was, visualize a third eye made of white light. Imagine that this eye is all-seeing. Take a moment to feel into this visualization.

Step 4: Now imagine radiating out from around this white eye a beautiful purple light—a sphere of this purple light radiating outward into the cosmos from your white light third eye. Imagine this purple light is all-encompassing, surrounding you in every direction. Cultivate a sense of spaciousness and limitlessness.

Step 5: Visualize five white lines of light extending out from your eye through this sphere of beautiful purple light into space, out into infinity. These five threads of light represent lines to potential futures. You may do more than five, but I find that five is usually about the right amount to have this sense of multiple potential futures. Really imagine these threads are reaching infinitely through this purple light out into the horizon, as far as you can imagine.

Step 6: Bring to mind any memories you are working with from the When You Have Felt This Before section. Focus on the feeling, not the content, of your imagination/insight/intuition memory. Allow this feeling to enhance your visual of your white third eye extending lines of light out into the purple light around you.

Step 7: Say the affirmations, cultivating the feeling of each as you do so:
> I am still.
> I am intuitive.
> I know things beyond words.
> I am imaginative.
> I have vision.
> I am wise.

Step 8: Rest in the feelings of openness, spaciousness, and future potential for as long as you like. Take your snapshot memory for quick reference later.

Step 9: When you're ready to move on from this Empowerment, dissolve the entire visual slowly in the reverse order from which you built it—the lines, the purple light, and the eye. Bring your attention back down to your belly. You may want to open your physical eyes at this point. Take five or more deep belly breaths focused on your belly so you're solidly back in your body and focused on physical reality before you move on.

Don't expect intuitive visions or imaginings during this exercise. In fact, if visions do start to occur while you're doing it, gently pull your mind back from them and refocus on the visualization step. If you are prone to visual intuition or thoughts, this may initially be difficult because activating your third eye through the Empowerment will stimulate it. What's important here is to gain control over your inner vision. Activating the Empowerment clears and generates the energy for all the functions of your third eye—imagination, insight, intuition, idea generation, and meditation. You will use this

Empowerment as you do the others—to activate your third eye energy *before* you engage in activities in which you need these functions.

When You Are Blocked

When our third eye is closed or its energies are not available to us, some of the issues are very similar to when we have a closed or weak sacral chakra. We feel stuck, trapped, or in a rut. We can't imagine any other life. However, with a blocked third eye we may feel *motivated* to change our lives but just can't see *how* to do it or even know what we want.

Indecisiveness is another common blocked third eye symptom because our intuition is inhibited. Without our intuition, we easily get stuck in mental wheel-spinning, weighing the pros and cons of every choice, shifting endlessly back and forth between options. Having no sense of intuition feels a little like walking in the dark—we don't have a sight line to guide us, so we put our hands out and grasp and feel for obstacles as we move along. We are so afraid that we will miss some crucial angle or piece of information that we become paralyzed in our search for a reason to pick one option over another.

In fact, a general overdependence on mental analysis is another common sign of a blocked third eye. Our ability to think and rationally analyze is a great tool, of course, and many decisions in life need to come from this intellectual perspective. But many others require insight—that other valuable third eye skill. When our third eye is weak, we don't have the needed insight to decide what is right for us or the ability to see deeply into any situation. We are stuck skimming along on the surface of our lives and the situations we find ourselves in. Mental analysis might feel like digging deeper, but in fact in some situations it keeps us stuck in self-referential paralysis.

We also may feel like others' motivations or feelings are a mystery to us. We may misread and misjudge others or feel confused by what they want from us. Our emotional intelligence is highly connected to our intuition and capacity for insight; without either, we may feel socially inept and boorish *or* appear that way to others but never recognize it ourselves.

Our imagination is limited when our third eye is blocked or weak, too— not only our ability to imagine new potential futures for ourselves but also creative thought altogether. We can't dream up new products or creatively problem solve. We can't put components together in a new way. We are stuck seeing and accepting the status quo, whether we like it or not. We may feel dissatisfied and long to imagine something different but can't, leaving us feeling frustrated and cut off.

On the other end of the spectrum of third eye dysfunction is the form of disassociation already mentioned—using spiritual and psychic experiences as a form of escapism. Someone may be constantly in communication with what they perceive to be angels, guides, or other spiritual forces but are so lost in communication with them that they have disconnected from their own lives. They may engage with spiritual practice as a means of escape instead of as a tool for growth.

Using the Third Eye

One of the most useful ways to use the Third Eye Empowerment in your day is when you have a decision to make and are feeling stuck. For example, say you are apartment hunting and need to decide which of two apartments to rent. You have run through all the pros and cons for each, talked it through with friends, and still cannot decide. Take some time out and activate the Third Eye Empowerment. Try not to think about the decision itself while you do so but after the affirmations and before you dissolve the visual, imagine yourself in each apartment. See if you notice a difference in feeling as you visualize yourself in each. Which feels better to you? Do you notice any change in your body as you imagine yourself in each one? Do you get a better sense of which one you actually want?

You can use this Empowerment with virtually any decision. It is more effective when you don't put pressure on yourself to make the decision on the spot right after the activation. Just engage in the exercise and add whatever you glean from it as another data point to consider. Often, a strong insight or intuition about what you should do will come to you later. The important thing is that you activate your third eye and link it to the decision you are trying to make. Doing so allows all levels of your being and psyche to process, and it loosens the grip of your mental spinning. You'll find that the best approach is to activate the third eye and then stop thinking about your decision, allowing your psyche and intuitive mind to work on it unhindered.

There are many other times throughout your day that you may want to activate the Third Eye Empowerment. Here are some ideas:

- When you are stuck on a problem. Activate the third eye, then let the problem go for a bit—take a walk or get involved with something else.
- Before you go into a brainstorming meeting or studio session *or* any time you want to generate ideas or create. You may want to combine this with the Sacral Lotus for inspiration.
- Before you interact with an individual or group for which you feel you need more insight. Perhaps you sense there is some undercurrent of emotion or politics that you can't quite grasp.
- Before you journal, engage in therapy, or explore another modality whose purpose is to face yourself or see something honestly about yourself.
- Whenever you are confused, feel foggy, or are caught in cycles of mental spinning.
- Before or while you are meditating, in prayer, or engaged in any activity you consider spiritual.

As for long-term work with the Third Eye Empowerment, of course the most common reason you might do so is to improve your intuition. Activating the Third Eye Empowerment daily will help by increasing how much you notice and process the energetic data coming into your energy body. Really, this is the starting point for any of us: increased *noticing*. We rarely need to increase our energetic *sensitivity*—the actual vibrations we are picking up—because there is so much we already pick up that we aren't paying attention to.

Counter to what you may think, activating your third eye doesn't generally increase your energetic sensitivity or trigger your "letting in" energies you don't want. You are already picking up all sorts of energies all of the time. Activating your third eye increases your ability to *process* these in a way that is useful for you. In fact, this actually helps with your energetic boundary setting and clearing because you become more aware of the energies you are coming into contact with. Often, we pick them up without noticing. Becoming more aware is an important step in improving how we care for and protect our energy body.

However, it is true that when we initially open our third eye chakra more, especially if it has been closed most of our life, we may at times feel as if we are taking in too much from the world. We need time to adjust as we adapt to processing all of the subtler stimuli we had been screening out. It also takes time to learn how to process this information into actual useful intuitions. We will cover more about energy protection and boundaries in the Second Skin chapter; for now, if you are working with the Third Eye Empowerment over a period of time specifically to increase your intuition, be mindful of how you are feeling. If you begin to feel spacey, ungrounded, overwhelmed by stimuli, or oversensitive, take a break for a few days. Working with the Second Skin, Root Bowl, and Navel Fire will also help, along with additional exercise or time in nature.

To utilize the Third Eye Empowerment to improve your intuition, activate it daily, pay special attention to thoughts that arise that may be intuitive, and do your best to validate them afterward. If, for example, you have the thought as you are looking for a parking space "If I turn left, I'll find one," then follow that thought and find out if it proves true. If you sense someone is lying to you, research and see if you can find if you were correct. If you find yourself thinking someone in your life may be feeling low, call them and see if it's so (and offer comfort, of course!). Experiment. Pay attention to thoughts that you may usually ignore and make an effort to test them.

Once you have been able to validate or invalidate such a thought—once you know whether or not you were correct—remember how the thought *felt* when it occurred to you. See if you can notice a difference between the feeling of the thought when you were correct and when you weren't. Developing the insight to begin to distinguish when a thought is being generated by your intuitive mind is the most important part of developing your intuition. When you are wrong, assess what might have affected your thinking—do you dislike the person you thought was lying and so were predisposed to think ill of them? Did you find a parking space to the left the two days before so your mind simply defaulted to that?

This kind of assessment draws upon our insight, one of those other third eye functions. As we've already discussed, developing your intuition goes hand in hand with developing your insight. The process may seem tedious at first but over time will become automatic.

Some forms of intuition can't really be validated, as they are based on trust. If you intuitively choose one apartment over another or one job over another, you may never know if you would have been happier with the other. Choosing to trust your intuition and allowing yourself to open to it as a valid method for helping you navigate your life isn't just about being "right"—it's about feeling true to yourself.

There are many other kinds of intuition besides what we've covered here. Some people receive information as visions, in dreams, through signs, through spirit communication, and several other ways. All are enhanced by working with the Third Eye Empowerment, and you can improve your ability to work with these other methods safely in the same way. It's beyond the scope of what I can do here to discuss these other methods, but I've provided my own favorite resources online. The point of the Chakra Empowerments is to help you use your chakras in daily life as opposed to full-scale psychic development.

There are many other reasons you may want to use the Third Eye Empowerment regularly for a period of time. Here are some examples:

- When you are trying to see a new direction for your life or open up to new potential futures.
- If you are trying to develop your imagination or are involved in a project that requires you to draw upon your imagination.
- If you feel you have a habit of being confused, foggy, or fuzzy that you would like to break.
- If you are in regular therapy and seeking deeper insight about yourself.

For all these purposes, just activate the Empowerment daily and let it go. Don't expect an epiphany or grand idea the moment you complete the process, although sometimes that may occur. Most of the time it is more like muscle conditioning—when you are looking to grow stronger, you don't expect it to happen with one workout. It takes time, and you should think in the same way when using the Third Eye Empowerment.

Women's Energetics: Reclaiming Intuition

Often the most relevant third eye work women must do is to release biases against our own intuition we have internalized as well as fears we have about using it. Intuition, and in particular women's intuition, has been demonized and denigrated in much the same way women's sexual energy has been. Historically this occurred first within religion, with the persecution of women who functioned as intuitive healers, astrologers, or general community guides. Then, with the rise of science, came an exultation of the rational mind and logical thinking, and a general disparagement or even disdain for intuitive thinking.

This denigration of intuition affects everyone, but contemporary women in particular have been affected the most deeply. Historical knowledge of the persecution of women for use of intuitive skills has negatively affected our relationship to our own intuition (and if you believe in past lives, karmic fears related to our own past persecution plays a role too). Then as women have joined organizational powers such as government and business in greater numbers we have done so mostly under the existing model, upholding rational modes of knowing as the most valid, and disavowing other forms. I find that women working in highly competitive and/or male-dominated industries (as I myself did for many years within the technology sector) are often less likely to engage in or affirm intuitive thinking as valid out of a fear of being perceived as flaky or ungrounded.

So, if you would like to improve your intuition through working with the Third Eye Empowerment or any of its other aspects, work on surfacing or releasing the biases you have internalized about it. As a child, was your intuition or imagination discouraged? Are you surrounded by people with whom you would be hesitant to discuss it? Do you fear being perceived as flaky, ungrounded, or unreliable if you engage with your third eye more? Does it feel unsafe to you? Identifying and releasing these biases and self-beliefs will help you to empower your third eye, and because it is one of the three chakras in your feminine pathway, it is essential to your ability to open to the power available through that Feminine Pathway Empowerment as well.

Skylar came to me at age twenty-nine to work on healing from sexual abuse she had experienced at the hands of her stepfather as a child. She was in an intensive psychic training program, and in our first session she listed all of the many workshops and modalities she had already engaged with in her search for healing. These included therapy, somatic therapy, yoga, EMDR, Reiki, acupuncture, shamanism, angel guidance, past life regression, various forms of meditation, and much more. She was a virtual encyclopedia of intuitive and healing methods, and had many stories of insights she had gleaned from this work.

However, Skylar had a hard time talking about any of her actual emotions or how her abuse affected her in her daily life. She tended to answer questions with a description of a psychic experience she had had in a workshop or healing session. She wanted to do the Sacral Lotus, as she had read about sacral chakra work on my website, which is what she felt she needed. When we activated it, she experienced visions and strong energetic sensations in her body, but I could not get her to connect with any emotions or energetic aspects of her sacral chakra itself.

I asked Skylar if in any of her healing work she had explored how she disassociated during abuse episodes of her childhood. This question shifted Skylar's entire demeanor. She had explored this in therapy and remembered that she had in fact "gone away" in her head whenever her stepfather came to her room to abuse her. She said she had gone away to mystical worlds, perhaps astral planes. I asked her how she felt in those worlds; "safe" was her answer.

Skylar began to realize she felt safer during mystic experience than in daily life. She was now willing to explore working with her third eye in a different way and focus on grounding. We worked with the third eye with the intention of developing insight, and with the Root Bowl and Sacral Lotus to connect her more deeply to her body and emotions. We focused on emotions Skylar experienced in daily life, especially patterns in her relationships with other people, something she tended to avoid. Skylar also decided to reenter therapy with a spiritual psychologist who honored her intuitive abilities. She is today a successful psychic in private practice and works with many women who themselves have experienced sexual trauma.

Skylar's story is an example of spiritual bypassing or spiritual disassociation—using spiritual, mystic, or healing experience or practice as a means for avoiding challenging emotions, relationships, or problems in daily life. The worlds that opened to her through her third eye had been her safe space during her abusive childhood and helped her survive it. It was only natural that she felt the most comfortable here and that she would seek out ways to recreate this safety. As Skylar began to work more emotionally, and with her lower chakras in particular, she was able to fully own her natural intuitive abilities and use them in the work she wanted to do in the world.

Sexual Trauma Healing: Grounding and Letting Go

Skylar's story highlights one of the main ways sexual trauma may affect a survivor's third eye chakra—creating a hyperdependence upon it. This behavior might involve disassociating through mystic experience (as in her case), or it might involve escaping into video games, movies, fantasy novels, or another medium that sends us to imaginary realms. In moderation, these are all marvelous third eye experiences, but if they become a way of avoiding real life, they hinder healing.

However, sexual trauma can also affect your third eye in the exact opposite way, by creating a fear of mystic, spiritual, or intuitive experience because it feels unsafe. This may manifest in part as patterns of hypervigilance, living in a state of heightened anxiety in which you are constantly scanning your surroundings for danger. This is especially common for survivors of surprise assaults or accidents. On the one hand, this state is grounded, in the sense that you are hyperaware of your body and the environment you are in. But that very hyperawareness makes it feel unsafe to engage in third eye activities such as daydreaming, imagination, or intuition. There is a gripping in the body based in anxiety that prevents opening and relaxing into your third eye.

In either case, working with your third eye as a sexual trauma survivor involves balancing a sense of safety and grounding with opening and letting go. It is about balance between your lower and upper chakras. Normally, I do not work with Third Eye Empowerment with sexual trauma survivors until we have spent a lot of time with the first three Empowerments, especially the Root Bowl. If you are complementing your healing with chakra work, it's especially important to spend time developing your lower chakras first before moving on to your third eye. Deep-seated patterns of either disassociation or hypervigilance will usually require talk therapy work in addition to energy work.

All this said, don't give up on your third eye. You deserve to experience all your energy body has to offer as well as all aspects of yourself, including your intuition. Reclaim this inner power, in a way and at a pace that feels safe and nurturing to you. Honor yourself for your bravery in doing so.

SEVEN
Crown Connection: Your Purpose

Related Chakras: Your seventh, or crown, chakra

Energies: Meaning, purpose, faith, hope, spirit, seeking, cosmic connection, divine union, grace, birth, death

Use For: Doubt, aimlessness, faithlessness, meaninglessness, disconnection, disillusionment, spiritlessness, spiritual dryness, isolation, mistrust

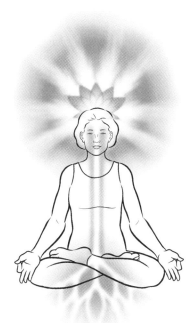

The crown chakra is our personal portal between spirit and ourselves, or, put another way, between our own individual spirit and the larger force of which we are a part. For you, that larger force might be God, Goddess, Allah, Yahweh, Brahman, Source, the Great Spirit, the universe, nature, nirvana, the Tao, the Divine, light, space, emptiness, interdependence, or nothing at all. These are words, and if there is one thing every religious and spiritual tradition tends to agree upon it's that a word in this case cannot capture in entirety what it refers to. We experience small bits and attempt to understand from there.

Our crown chakra is our intermediary in this process. It connects us to the vastness that we cannot completely comprehend. This chakra provides the connection point for experiences we can then translate into our mind as spiritual or mystic. Unlike other chakras, this one is both in and out of our body—halos, those golden or white discs around a figure's head found in religious art around the world, are representations of it. Indeed, the chakra's location reflects its dual role, a bridge between our individual physical self and the beyond, as it is located both inside and above the rear top part of our head, where our rear fontanel is when we are born.

When we are born, our skull has two places where it is not fused shut, in order to allow for birth and the fast growth of our brain in our infant stage. Both places are called fontanels; the rear one, located right where the top of our skull starts to slope downward toward the back, closes first (at two or three months old). This closure corresponds in time to our first tiny shift toward energetic autonomy from our parents and caretakers.

During gestation and before this fontanel closes, we have little sense of separation from spirit or anyone physical around us. We experience one big, vast energy and spiritual field. In some ways, we could say the spiritual growth process is one of reestablishing this connection. Not every religion conceives of the spiritual process in the same way, of course, but the similarities in mystics' descriptions of their experiences across all different cultures and traditions is astonishing; they also tie very closely to the main chakras we have covered, particularly the sacral, heart, third eye, and crown. Descriptions of light, surges of energy, and feelings of union or grace within these chakras are universal. These experiences are not just confined to formal spiritual practice either—we may have them out in nature, when viewing art, when engaged in sex, or during many other activities.

Within these experiences, the crown is about union and dissolution. Practices within some energy-based traditions involve consciously bringing energy up from the root chakra to the crown for the purposes of initiating this union and dissolution, the upward pathway introduced in chapter 4. Other spiritual practices involve merging the root and crown energy into the heart or entering into source through the inner doorway of any chakra. While not all traditions use the word "chakra," the chakras are nevertheless a mapping system through which we can understand these experiences.

Does working with your crown have to be exclusively about spirituality if you don't resonate with it? Not necessarily. The crown chakra within our daily lives is about our search for *meaning*, the foundation for our sense of purpose and faith. It is the energy of hope. While our third eye helps us to see future potentials, our crown is the energy of hope that infuses and animates these ideas; it is the energy behind our search for answers to life's big questions.

The crown is also linked to birth and death. Some cultures believe that our soul enters and leaves the body through the fontanel at birth and death, and that we can travel beyond and through it when we are alive. Whether or not it is literally an entrance or exit point, an open crown chakra is linked to our awareness of our own mortality. We are aware of the transience of our physical body and the effect of time upon it. Through our crown we sense both that we are—and are more than—this form.

The most important feature of our crown chakra is its relationship to our own direct experience and inner quest. It is not about the beliefs or philosophies we have adopted from authority figures or institutions. We may be introduced to either spiritual beliefs or other kinds of ideologies that are meaningful to us through authority figures such as parents, teachers, religious leaders, political leaders, and so on, but they become our own when we move beyond simply accepting them blindly, adopting them due to our own questioning and experience.

Mikaela described herself as feeling burnt out and aimless in her work. She had wanted to be a teacher since she was ten, and had been excited to be hired as a ninth grade Social Studies teacher straight out of college. But after two years in this role, she was not enjoying it and had begun to doubt that she was doing any good. She was fed up with the bureaucracy involved, the limits on her lesson plans, the demands of parents, and the disinterest of her students. She was disillusioned by her fellow teachers, many of whom she felt were just phoning it in.

I asked Mikaela if she wanted to change schools or careers. She said she didn't know; there wasn't anything else in particular she felt passionate about. I also asked her about hobbies and relationships. She liked to hike and had a lot of friends she hung out with regularly but there weren't any romantic interests at the moment, and she didn't feel very excited about any of it. She had worked for a long time to have the life she had but was now questioning the value of all of it. She did not exhibit signs of depression per se, but she was definitely not happy.

We began with the Crown Connection to increase the energies of hope and purpose and help Mikaela to cut through the feeling of meaninglessness and aimlessness she currently felt. I asked her to do the Crown Connection daily between sessions and to try to determine what she most valued in her life through a series of questions. What were the most important personal attributes a person could have to her? Who did she admire? What did she believe in? What experiences did she most want to have in life? What experiences currently brought her joy?

Mikaela reported having a tough time with these questions early in the week but did feel like doing the Crown Connection beforehand helped her with them as the week progressed. The hardest question for her was, "What do you believe in?" She felt she believed in education and had wanted to be a part of that, but her disillusionment at work caused her to start thinking that was naïve. She did not connect with the idea of belief beyond that. She told me she had been raised in a very strict church but had rejected it as an adult. The pastor had been accused of mismanagement, and she believed the entire community had been hypocritical, including her parents. It was a huge source of contention between them, although they had decided to put it behind them and never spoke about religion anymore.

I asked Mikaela if she missed anything about being part of her childhood church. She responded that she missed the sense of community and belonging, as well as the practice of regular prayer and the sense of spiritual connection it provided. I asked her if she prayed now or ever felt that sense of connection on her own. She felt she did not want to pray, that it was the purview of her childhood church; she expressed feeling too disillusioned to partake in that anymore. But she did say that being in nature on hikes, especially longer hikes into remote regions, was the closest she got to the same feeling as in prayer. For her, nature offered a spiritual experience.

We worked more with the Crown Connection, and I asked Mikaela to consider visiting other churches or communities, reading some spiritual books, and/or experimenting with prayer on her own. I suggested she consider herself a *seeker* rather than a *believer* for a time—give herself permission to explore rather than adopt a particular faith. I also encouraged her to join a hiking group or make that a more formal part of her life. We then also activated the Third Eye Empowerment and sought to envision more potential future directions for her.

Over time, Mikaela worked with both the Crown Connection and Third Eye Empowerments, as well as with others to heal some of the wounds and blocks that had developed through these two disillusionments in her life—first her religion, then the career goal she'd had for so long. She began to construct her own sense of what she valued and felt meaningful to her, and she began to feel more excited about options for her life. She explored meditation and began to read books on different types of spirituality. She planned a trip through several national parks with friends and became interested in environmentalism. She proposed an environmentally themed service project as an after-school activity at her school, and to her excitement, it was approved and many students were interested. Although she still wasn't sure if she would stay with teaching long-term, she reconnected to a sense of meaning and purpose in her life.

Disillusionment is a major blow to our crown chakra. When a person, organization, or belief system we have admired or relied upon for a long time lets us down, we can spiral quickly into feelings of meaninglessness and aimlessness. We all live our lives based on certain values and principles, conscious or not, that determine our goals and shape our identity. When they fail us, we flounder. However, we do not always have to know exactly what we believe; as in Mikaela's case, sometimes we just need to open ourselves to asking, considering ourselves a seeker. Then we can approach life with curiosity and explore with openness what will provide us value and purpose.

When You Have Felt This Before

If you engage in spiritual practice—meditation, prayer, religious ritual, song, sacred art making, and so on—and it triggers for you a sense of connection to the Divine (however you define that), you have experienced the energy of your crown chakra in that form. Often these experiences involve much more than our crown; they can feel like whole-body and whole-energy-body experiences. Our heart and third eye in particular may light up. There are many kinds and levels of these experiences, and spiritual texts in all the major religions offer maps and descriptions, but all involve the crown to some extent.

You may also have felt this same kind of experience in nature, when viewing art, during intimacy with a partner, or through other activities that felt sacred to you and brought you out of yourself. When you feel a sense of being lifted, or united, with your environment, other people, or a greater force, your crown energy is activated and flowing in some way.

If you have given birth or witnessed a birth or peaceful death, you may have felt the energy of your crown chakra in those moments. An opening occurs in the individual being birthed or dying, and it often triggers an opening in our own crown chakra in response. This includes witnessing the birth and death of animals if they are peaceful. (Witnessing a fatal accident or difficult birth or death does not generally have this effect, as we don't feel safe enough for our crown to open.) If you have such a memory, tap into it and see if you can identify the crown chakra feeling. It can be difficult to tease it out from whatever emotions you were feeling at the time, so focus your memory on the feeling in and around your head.

If you have ever received an idea that filled you with purpose and perhaps felt like it was being given to you (like a divine download), this experience is also an example of crown chakra energy. If the crown is involved, there is a real sense of purpose and meaning associated with whatever idea you are having—that is, it feels like you were born to do it or you must manifest it to give your life purpose. It feels like a turning point in your life.

When you are involved in very active seeking, spiritually or ideologically—when you are in a phase of life in which you are digging deep to discover meaning—your crown is very active. This might be a day in which you feel particularly inspired, or it might be a phase of your life in which you are searching in this way. We sometimes have opening periods in our lives during which we sense something new on the horizon but aren't quite sure what it is and are driven to find out. Although this search is often spiritual in nature, it isn't always; what's most salient here is that it feels important to us, and central to our being.

If you have had any of these experiences in your life, consider journaling about them to recall what you felt in more detail. The crown is subtle; reconnecting with what you felt there may take some time but can be very helpful when you are working to activate the Crown Connection. I find that people tend to think they can't activate the Crown Connection when they want to, like it's a gift they have to wait for or spontaneous grace. But you absolutely can activate your crown whenever you like, whenever you need more of its energies in your being.

Activation Steps

This Empowerment is called Crown *Connection* because it is about connecting your crown energies with your body. It is designed to open your crown and help you bring down insights, ideas, and experiences into your mind, psyche, and body. It is not a meditation practice per se, where we would seek to experience a divine state. As with all the Empowerments in this book, this one is oriented around how you may use your crown energies in your daily life, within a day and for longer term growth.

As always, prepare your space, files, notes, and visual before you begin.

> *Step 1:* Sit with your spine aligned, place your hand on your navel, and take several deep breaths to connect with your physical body.

> *Step 2:* Bring your awareness to this closed fontanel on the rear top part of your head. Feel where your skull begins to slope downward here.

Hold your hand, open and palm down, one or two inches above this part of your head. For several breaths, imagine you are reaching your awareness up and out the top of your head, trying to reach your hand.

Step 3: Put your hand down; where your hand was, visualize a beautiful, radiant lotus. Yes, we're using the lotus again, just as we did with the Sacral Lotus Empowerment. This lotus is open, luminous, and made of gold and silver light. The bottom of it is resting right at the top of your head, but the petals are rising up out of your head, radiating a halo of gold light around you.

Step 4: Imagine that you are slowly bringing gold and silver light down from this lotus, straight down the middle of your body. It moves down the center of your head, even with your third eye, down through your neck behind your throat chakra, down through your heart chakra, down through your stomach and your navel chakra, down through your sacral chakra and your pelvis, all the way down to your tailbone. From there it reaches down into the earth, and it sprouts roots in the earth.

Step 5: Hold this visual for two to three minutes. Focus on the open, radiant quality of the flower, and the strong connection all the way through you down into the earth. It is like you are planting the lotus in your being, and the earth beneath you. If your mind wanders, repeat the process of visualizing the lotus and imagining light coming all the way down your body and rooting into the earth.

Step 6: Now bring to mind any When You Have Felt This Before memories you would like to use to affirm the feeling of your crown.

Step 7: Say your affirmations, really trying to feel them as true as you do:
I find meaning in my life.
I feel part of something larger than myself.
I have faith.
I am connected.
I know my purpose in this moment.

Step 8: Dissolve this visual. Bring your hands back to your belly, taking a few deep belly breaths in your body to ground.

The lotus is symbolic of spiritual awakening because it is a flower that floats beautifully on the top of the water, while underneath, its stalk reaches deep into the mud of a pond or river. It represents a union of the muddy reality of our life and the transcendent beauty and light of realization. With the Crown Connection we are not seeking to escape our lives, but to bring the energy of union and meaning connected to our crown into our daily lives.

When You Are Blocked

Like Mikaela, when your crown chakra is blocked or weak, you may feel aimless and directionless. You may feel that your life lacks meaning or purpose. Often a disappointment or disillusionment triggers this state. Perhaps some person you admired or a goal you had sought did not turn out to be what you thought it would be. Sometimes we feel this way after something we have looked forward to for a long time—we have been waiting for a big event; now it is over, and we crash.

Sometimes we self-medicate this state of purposelessness by creating one goal or event after another for ourselves so that we always have something in the future on which we are pinning our hopes. I once had a coworker who started planning her next vacation every year as soon as the last was complete, and she would spend hours each week researching every decision, while daydreaming and talking constantly about her next trip. While there is nothing wrong with planning and excitement, we are not connected to the present when our entire focus is the future. Whether living for your next vacation, promotion, or the next weekend, you won't be grounded in your body and life if this is habitual. From an energetic perspective, a certain amount of crown energy *is* activated through this constant focus on the future—there is a sense of purpose—but it is only skin deep and distracts us from the deeper work of using our crown energy to build a life based on meaning and purpose.

A stereotypical midlife crisis often has elements of this kind of crown self-medication and distraction. As someone faces their waning youth and realizes that they have not achieved what they had thought they would by a certain age, they may distract themselves through dramatic purchases or changes in their life that are not actually tied to a deeper soul search of what matters to them. However, there actually is a huge opportunity at this time to engage in deep seeking and let go of old goals and values that no longer feel authentic in order to create a life that reflects a new foundation for meaning.

We may experience a similar break with meaning or faith after a big loss in our lives—the loss of a loved one through death, a divorce or breakup, or even the loss of a job. Once we have moved through our grief, the hole left in our lives may lead to this feeling of meaninglessness. If our loss has been through death, we may also be facing our own mortality in a new way, and questioning the value of our life from that perspective.

A loss of religious or spiritual faith, a deep questioning of principles we once held dear, or an inability to feel a connection to a spiritual power in the way we have in the past are all tied to a weak or blocked crown chakra. Sometimes called a dark night of the soul, a deep spiritual crisis can become the ground for a powerful deepening of our spiritual understanding. To do so, we must reengage as a seeker to actively pursue new knowledge and look deeply inward, all of which will engage our crown.

It's worth noting that this kind of spiritual crisis is very different from a kundalini crisis. Kundalini is one form of energy that moves through the chakras; it is the primary energy of spiritual growth, and its rise into the crown is a natural part of spiritual experience and realization. We are not working explicitly with kundalini in this book, although it will naturally be activated whenever you work with any chakra, particularly the crown. A kundalini crisis occurs when someone's energy body becomes overwhelmed by the amount of kundalini moving through the chakras that is triggered by formal kundalini practice or possibly spontaneously. A crown chakra crisis is more about loss of *meaning* than energetic overwhelm. While working through a kundalini crisis involves smoothing and grounding your energy body, a crown chakra spiritual crisis involves engaging your curiosity and sense of wonder to actively *seek*—and thereby open—your crown to new information and experience.

Anytime you experience paralyzing doubt, whether about yourself or some aspect of your life, it's a sign your crown is affected. It's important to distinguish between healthy questioning and skepticism and debilitating self-doubt or paralysis. Healthy questioning is actually an expression of a strengthened crown chakra because it represents seeking; it is part of the search for truth and meaning. A search has direction and an opening quality to it, while paralyzing doubt has a directionless or closed quality. Understanding the difference is key to understanding how our crown energy can help us move forward, and how a lack of it can immobilize us. An open crown chakra is not about blind faith, nor about shutting down questioning, it is about questioning that is truly rooted in a search for meaning.

Using the Crown Connection

As you can probably tell by the description of how crown chakra blocks manifest, the crown chakra is more of a big picture chakra. Working with the Crown Connection therefore is usually more relevant for phases of our life as opposed to particular daily events. Nevertheless, there are daily situations or times in which we may want to activate the Crown Connection. Here are some examples:

- Before meditation, prayer, spiritual art-making, ritual, or any other practice you consider spiritual.
- Before or while experiencing nature or art, to help you connect to these in a deeper way.
- When reading a spiritual, philosophical, or ideological book in which you are engaged as part of a search for meaning.
- When feeling too caught up in the minutia of your life with no sense of the larger value or meaning.
- When involved in activities related to manifesting a goal directly linked to a larger purpose or value you hold in your life.
- When witnessing a birth or death so that you may connect spiritually to the experience.

As for long-term growth, the main phases of your life in which you will want to use the Crown Connection are those in which you are seeking to redefine or reclaim meaning; as we have already established, this is very often after a crisis of some type. For example:

- When working through a deep disappointment or disillusionment.
- After the loss of a loved one or another kind of loss that leaves a hole in your life.
- During a crisis of faith.
- During a midlife crisis.
- After a shock or trauma that has shaken your sense of safety or trust.
- When you are feeling lost, aimless, or purposeless.

It's important to note that in any of these cases, your crown may not be the first chakra you work with. You need to make sure you are stable before you engage regularly with your crown. You may need to work with your root or heart first for example, in order to ground yourself, address anxiety, or support your initial grieving process. You can begin to work with the Crown Connection regularly when you are ready to question and examine your experience, with the purpose of determining what you value.

Any phase of questioning may also be a time you want to work with the Crown Connection regularly. For example:

- When you are actively seeking answers to life's big questions (e.g., through a spiritual or ideological quest).
- When you are entering into a retreat or deep spiritual practice.
- When you are reexamining your values and purpose or seeking new ones.
- When you feel you have become disconnected from your spirituality; perhaps you feel you've hit a plateau in your growth or lost your sense of belief.
- When you are experiencing a lot of self-doubt, or doubt in general.

Claudia was a long-time yoga practitioner and popular instructor who had studied with a well-known teacher within an international organization for almost thirty years. She had her own yoga studio, traveled widely to teach yoga retreats, and often attended retreats herself. Her yoga lineage was very much her spiritual path; she credited it with helping her heal from depression and migraines as well as moving on from a difficult childhood to creating a happy, heart-centered life for herself. She had seen yoga benefit many of her students as well; in fact, I had first met her at a retreat she taught which I attended.

When Claudia contacted me many years later, it was because she was struggling to make sense of a recent sex scandal that had rocked the yoga organization of which she was a part. The founder, of whom Claudia had been one of the first Western students, had recently resigned amid a gradually increasing onslaught of accusations of sexual harassment, abuse, and assault by many female students. The organization was crumbling, Claudia's own studio was losing students, and she herself was devastated. She had held this man in high esteem and considered him her primary spiritual guide.

Claudia felt simultaneously angry, duped, grief-stricken, and culpable—had she missed something? Had she turned a blind eye? Some of the women who had come forward were her friends but had never told her what had happened. When she asked them why, they told her they didn't think she would believe them, as she was so close to their teacher. At the same time, she did not know what to think of the man she had believed in for so long, the man whom she had modeled her own spiritual path after in many ways. If he was an abuser and liar, what did that say about his teachings? What was real and what was deception? Was the life she had built for herself based on delusion? Had she spent all these years perpetuating harm while she thought she was doing good?

There was a lot to unpack in Claudia's situation. We first worked with her root and heart to help ground and soothe her. Claudia was having difficulty eating and sleeping (in a crisis like this, the crown is not the first chakra to work with). As she stabilized, we began working with the Crown Connection and establishing a way for Claudia to sort through the many questions she was grappling with. She realized the biggest blow was the doubt that had been triggered for her about the yoga teachings upon which she had built her life. Her questioning of the validity of these had shaken her to her core; where she would normally turn to teachings for guidance as well as the yoga practice in times of need, she now found it difficult.

Claudia decided to work with the Crown Connection daily with the goal of strengthening her direct spiritual connection. She followed this by a period of journaling in which she consciously reviewed times in her life in which a practice or teaching had helped her. She sought to verify each teaching through her *own* experiences and disconnect them from her teacher. Eventually she realized that although she had had many personal experiences of the teachings helping her, she had never separated the teachings *from* her teacher. In a way, she had never truly acknowledged what she learned as her own. As she let go of her projections about him and the sense that her spiritual path was dependent upon having him as her intermediary, her own faith in the teachings was actually strengthened. She also spent time healing her own hurt and releasing the feelings of shame and self-blame she held around the entire situation.

With time, Claudia healed and flourished and was able to play a key role in helping others in her yoga community work through their disillusionment. She reconstructed her own studio around the teachings that resonated the most for her, personally, adding some things from her own direct experience and her personal journey. Her life and business began to thrive again, and Claudia felt that as painful as the entire experience had been, she had actually come into her personal and spiritual power in an entirely new way because of it.

Claudia experienced a disillusionment that shook the very foundation upon which she had built her life. She had to reexamine everything in order to determine for herself what was of value, what she knew to be beneficial, and what was not. She had to rely on her own direct spiritual connection rather than a spiritual authority or organization. Although this process stripped her down in difficult ways, she emerged ultimately stronger and more spiritually connected than ever. This is the opportunity of spiritual crisis and disillusionment in general. Our crown chakra energies empower our ability to navigate these situations based on our own direct spiritual connection.

Women's Energetics: Direct Connection

Claudia's story (and to some extent, Mikaela's) demonstrates one of the main ways a woman's crown chakra may be blocked or compromised—allowing spiritual or ideological framework to become dependent upon an outside authority or intermediary. And although it's not always the case, most often the intermediary or authority is male.

All the world's major religious and spiritual traditions have been male-dominated for the majority of recorded history. While there have been many powerful women mystics throughout the centuries within all these traditions (in addition to female-centric traditions outside of these major ones), the whole of history notes religious and spiritual leadership to be the purview of men, as it has been with political, business, and cultural leadership. In many ways, there has been more focus in recent decades on breaking down barriers for women within all the other arenas combined than within the religious and spiritual leadership arena. This is changing these days, but the process is slow. In the meantime, the resulting belief from centuries of women internalizing the message that we are spiritually second-class citizens, runs very deep.

Our capacity to directly connect to spirit (whatever that means to you and in whatever form) is fundamental to our humanity; it's wired into our brains, just as it is into our energy body—through our crown chakra. When we internalize the message that we are not supposed to connect directly on our own but instead must do so through a male religious leader, teacher, or even a male body, it shuts down our direct connection. Our crown chakra is essentially blocked or only able to open to the extent that our male intermediary allows us to connect or that we allow ourselves.

Complicating this situation is the reality of sexual abuse and harassment within these institutions as well as the pain, disempowerment, and disillusionment that result from these experiences. These feelings can cause someone to shut down their spiritual connection entirely. To be clear: It's not only men who abuse power, nor are victims always women—and certainly not all men abuse their power in this way. There are unfortunately plenty of women sexual abusers and plenty of male victims. As well, there has been and is an abundance of authentic and spiritually pure male teachers. The point is that in our current period of intense reckoning regarding the male abuse of power over women, the headlines have been increasingly—but only recently—about the downfall of powerful men about whom the truth has finally surfaced regarding their long-standing abuse of women. While those who make the news tend to be in business or political leadership positions, there has also been a steady stream of such stories within religious and spiritual communities.

What we are experiencing now is a reckoning and rebalancing—a painful but necessary one. It has left many women severely disillusioned about religion and spirituality. Some have turned to female-dominated traditions or female teachers or leaders. Others, like Mikaela in the first story shared in this chapter, have thrown it all aside. It's not my place to say what is right for you, but what I can say is that I feel, from both my own experience and that of the many women I have worked with, that finding female spiritual role models and stories both historical and contemporary is extremely important for women seekers at this time in history. I don't mean that you cannot have a male teacher, priest, reverend, or spiritual counselor—what I'm talking about is the importance of actively seeking out the feminine as well as models for the feminine connection to spirit.

Why is it important to seek out the feminine? Conditioning runs deep, and when it comes to the crown chakra, we can in fact *block ourselves* from spiritual connection based on our subtle conditioning. We may feel, as Claudia did, that we have fully owned our own spiritual path, internalized and authenticated the teachings or belief system we've received, and connected directly. And yet, we may be holding ourselves back, often in a subtle way. We seek permission and authentication from the male religious authorities in our lives. Patterns of emotional codependency, unworthiness, or the need for a father figure are all part of this conditioning too.

I myself have been a lifelong spiritual seeker and have been fortunate to have both wonderful male and female teachers in this lifetime, all of whom have empowered me to seek and experience my own spiritual insight and connection. I went through a phase of rejecting the idea of "women's spirituality," as it felt too divisive to me. I remember thinking at the time that surely spirit and spiritual realization were beyond gender, right? What I eventually decided for myself is that they certainly *are* beyond gender, but the path—the challenges we face in connecting directly to the Divine or our own inner wisdom—is often gender specific, at least at this time in history. Men and woman face many different obstacles, and as we work through them, feminine role models and stories are essential.

As I hope I've made a case for by now, part of what distinguishes our journeys are the differences in our energy bodies, and the particular types of blocks we encounter. Most blocks to the crown chakra are not gender-specific, but the *seeking* aspect of the crown is what connects it to the masculine energy pathway of the root/navel/throat/crown chakras. All of these chakras, in their default expression, are outward reaching, including this seeking side of the crown—it is a reaching outward in our search for meaning and purpose. To the extent the masculine pathway has been the purview of men, and the feminine pathway of women (denigrated, to boot), our right to spiritual and religious connection (crown) has been oppressed, as much as our right to our bodies (root), power in the world (navel), and voice (throat) have been. As we work toward owning our entire masculine energy pathway, we contribute to a wider energetic shift.

Sexual Trauma Healing: Rebuilding Self-Faith

If you have been abused or assaulted by a spiritual or religious leader or mentor in your life, male or female, then part of your healing work is looking at how your own spirituality has been affected. Has your disillusionment with this individual caused you to reject all spirituality, or the entirety of the tradition they were part of? Are there any parts of it you wish to reexamine? Are there aspects you miss? It is essential to do the work to distinguish what is authentically spiritually "yours" (via teachings or guidance you believe are valid) from the corrupted actions of your abuser or assaulter. You may be able to reclaim parts of your experience that are meaningful to you and integrate them into your life.

It is not always abuse by a spiritual or religious leader that can undermine a survivor's faith in spirituality. Sometimes it is lack of protection from a loved one who is religious. One survivor I know had a very religious mother who knew she was being abused but did not stop it. This caused this survivor to reject all religion and spirituality as hypocrisy. The wounds of betrayal and mistrust are not confined to those caused directly by your abuser or assaulter.

Work you do to surface and heal these wounds is part of your healing journey, and chakra work can aid you in this process.

Consider too how your overall faith in *yourself* may have been shaken. This is another variation on the shame and self-blame patterns we spoke about in the Sacral Lotus chapter. Often when our abuser or assaulter is someone we trusted, especially if we were a teen or adult when the abuse or assault took place, it shakes our faith in ourselves to judge others. This in turn undermines our faith in our intuition and spiritual experiences. Working to rebuild your own faith in yourself is a big part of the process if you are a sexual trauma survivor activating your Third Eye Empowerment and Crown Connection.

Of course, as with the third eye, crown chakra blocks can be on the opposite end of the spectrum—instead of spiritual experience being blocked, there may be patterns of disassociation involved, seeking mystic experience or guidance as a distraction or escape from deeper pain. Grounding is particularly important for bringing forth the insight necessary to see such patterns. Because this particular crown Chakra Empowerment focuses on the downward path and grounds your open crown energy in your body and other chakras, it rarely magnifies this kind of spiritual disassociation and can play a role in helping you to develop the discernment required to sort out what is realization and what is escape.

EIGHT
Second Skin: Your Boundary

Related Chakras: Your root (first) and navel (third) chakras

Energies: Protection, energetic integrity, boundaries, strength, stamina, endurance, resilience

Use For: Lack of boundaries, feeling unprotected, taking on others' emotions, fatigue, social anxiety, comfort eating, or for energetic boundaries and endurance

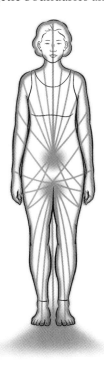

Many women find this chapter's Empowerment the most useful and life-transforming. The Second Skin provides an energetic filter and boundary that helps us maintain our energetic integrity and prevents us from taking on the emotions or negativity of others. As we've discussed, there are historical, cultural, and energetic factors that influence how we manage our energy. Women tend to prioritize others' emotions over their own energetic integrity and often take on others' emotional energy as a result. Meanwhile, because our energy body is centripetal by default and linked so deeply to the receptive sacral chakra and the feminine pathway of the sacral, heart, and third eye, we tend to pull energies in unconsciously and neglect to put down boundaries for ourselves as needed. If you have been sexually abused or assaulted, then your most fundamental boundary, that of your body, was violated against your will, and that leaves a lasting imprint that may also undermine your sense that you can or have a right to enforce boundaries.

As should be clear by now, all the Chakra Empowerments initially function on an energetic level that, with repetition, can manifest shifts on a psychological level that fundamentally change your way of being in the world. Perhaps no Empowerment has a greater potential for this shift than the Second Skin. If you feel you have had trouble owning your right to take up space in the world and insisting upon others honoring it, working with the Second Skin can be the Empowerment you need to change this once and for all. At some point, activating it will become second nature, your normal state of being rather than something you have to consciously activate.

Working with the Second Skin will also help you to let go of any artificial means of creating boundaries that you may have adopted or ways you are self-medicating when your boundaries are violated. These may be interpersonal patterns of pushing people away through anger or abrasiveness that have felt like your only recourse for feeling protected. Or it may be patterns of eating comfort foods and/or holding on to excess weight in attempts to mute the pain of boundary violation when it occurs, or to create a physical buffer between yourself and others. We all have artificial methods of self-protection, but most of them don't work. It is only when we truly feel capable of controlling which energies enter our being that we are able to let go of the need for many of these methods.

Notice that I said "controlling which energies enter our being," and not "controlling which energies we come into contact with." This is a very important distinction. I find that often when someone comes to me wanting to work on energetic boundaries, what they actually want is for me to assure them there is a way to guarantee nothing bad will ever happen to them or that they can manifest a life in which they will encounter no negativity. This desire is perfectly understandable—feeling safe and secure is our most fundamental need; especially if you have experienced trauma in your life, you may feel desperate for a way to feel safe in the world. The Second Skin will provide this, but not by controlling your world. Instead, it helps you prevent negative energy from entering your being when you encounter it, and it strengthens your resilience in the face of it.

The Second Skin is close to you, right on top of your skin; it's not like a deflective bubble. A bubble separates you from the world, while the Second Skin keeps you connected to it, and in fact can help you improve your intuition because it allows you to sense energies more clearly, rather than blindly absorbing them. As a filter, it helps you to choose what gets in and what doesn't. The Second Skin really is a tool for empowering your awareness and choice within your daily life. It's not about turning outward for protection—it is about standing in your own power and tapping into your own discernment and resilience. When we do this, we emanate the message that we are not to be tampered with or taken advantage of—and yes, this often does affect how people treat us. We are protected from the outside, though not in a knight-in-shining-armor kind of way.

As part of working with the Second Skin, we will also begin to talk more about the cycles and phases of our feminine energy body, including how it shifts during menstruation, pregnancy, and menopause. Living in women's bodies, we have very definite cycles and phases, and our energy bodies will shift in accordance. This means we may need to work with the Second Skin differently at various times—and we will cover this in the Women's Energetics section of this chapter.

Toni came to me as part of a larger health transformation she was seeking. She had struggled with her weight her entire life, and at the age of thirty-one had found out she was prediabetic. Her doctor had told her it was essential she lose weight, so she had embarked on a medically supported weight loss plan that included counseling to get to the root of any contributing emotional eating patterns. Toni was very spiritual, a long-time meditator and student of astrology and energy healing modalities, so she also wanted to explore ways she could support her life changes energetically.

Although Toni was already aware that she was an emotional eater, through her counseling she had come to realize just how much her eating was tied to social anxiety. She was so sensitive to others' moods that she was on edge in most interactions. She would feel anxious or off-balance at the slightest negativity expressed by anyone, even if it wasn't directed at her. Any sign of conflict between people or unhappiness or displeasure in a group when she was present would trigger feelings of stress and her being person-ally responsible. She would expend energy trying to shift the mood, but it would leave her drained. If someone directed a criticism her way or exhibited even a slight sign of displeasure with anything she said or did, she could be upset for days and even lose sleep over the encounter. She used food, espe-cially carbohydrate-filled comfort foods, as a buffer before, and for soothing after, such encounters.

I worked with several Empowerments with Toni to support her but most of our work was with the Second Skin. Toni was a classic empath in the way she absorbed others' emotions into her own body, and carrying extra weight was substituting as an energetic boundary for her. I asked Toni to activate the Sec-ond Skin every morning before leaving the house, and to activate it frequently throughout her day, especially before any meetings or group encounters.

Over the coming weeks, Toni began to realize the roots of her empathic tendencies. Her father had left her family when she was eight, and her mother had fallen into a depression from which she had never fully recovered. As the oldest of three children, Toni had assumed responsibility for all of them at this young age. Because her mother often had phases where she was upset by the slightest bickering amongst her siblings, Toni grew especially sensitive to any discord and took personal responsibility for it. She also tried to take on her mother's pain to heal her and her younger siblings' unhappiness to soothe them. She developed patterns of taking on everyone's emotions for them, never asserting her own needs or boundaries. Instead, she turned to food.

Through these insights, her new health routine, and diligent activation of the Second Skin, Toni began to shift her way of being in the world. As soon as she sensed her anxiety rising in a social setting or her tendency to begin to take responsibility for someone's mood, she would affirm the Second Skin on the spot and settle back into a feeling of energetic autonomy and strength. She would also use the Second Skin whenever she had a craving for carbs that she knew was rooted in stress from this empathic pattern.

With time and discipline, Toni lost the weight she needed to lose and created entirely new eating and exercise routines. But for her, even more importantly, she successfully shifted her energetic default. She no longer went out into the world feeling responsible for everyone else's moods or taking on their negativity. She therefore no longer needed extra weight as a buffer or carbs to self-medicate her anxiety. She felt resilient and clear in her own body, and she knew how to re-center herself in this feeling whenever she felt triggered.

Of course, weight loss is not simply a matter of developing energetic boundaries; you should always consult a health care practitioner regarding your weight and any diet you embark upon. For our purposes here, energy absorption is one of many reasons we may crave food when we don't need it, especially comfort-food carbs. Eating these foods can be a form of self-medication, and the resulting extra weight can create an artificial sense of energetic boundary. Getting to the root of our emotional eating and developing true boundaries through Second Skin can help us to shift this pattern.

Activation Steps

Second Skin is our first multi-Chakra Empowerment. As such, memories of When You Have Felt This Before are less relevant, so I won't devote a section to it in the remaining chapters. However, because the Second Skin combines the root and navel chakra energies, you may want to draw upon memories related to those chakras. Just to review, here are some examples of when you may have felt each component chakra's energies:

- *Root:* when surrounded by people with whom you feel safe and trusting; when engaged in activities that make you feel strong and present in your physical body; when feeling connected to nature; when feeling fully present and grounded in a moment.

- *Navel:* when you have achieved a goal through personal effort; when engaged in activities that you know you are good at; when drawing upon your determination and willpower; when focused and executing tasks with precision; when you were able to pull back and objectively assess a situation.

Standing is often the best position in which to activate the Second Skin, but once you have learned it you will be able to activate it from any position. Take a strong stance, with your feet hip-distance apart, ideally with feet flat on the ground or floor without shoes. Standing in this manner will help you feel as if you are really drawing upon the earth's energy to empower your root and navel chakras. If you are not able to stand, find a sitting position in which your feet are firmly touching the ground if possible.

Step 1: Assume your strong stance—feet hip-width apart, feet connected to the floor. Breathe into your belly as you do at the start of activating the other Empowerments, but this time *really* focus on your connection to the floor and beneath you to the earth.

Step 2: After a few breaths, bring your awareness to your root chakra at your tailbone. Just as you do when activating the Root Bowl, imagine vibrant red light flowing up from the earth to support you, and empowering a red sphere of light at your tailbone. Visualize this red sphere of light growing brighter and bringing a sense of physical vitality and strength to your physical body.

Step 3: Now visualize a matching red sphere of light just below your navel, where you would visualize your Navel Fire when activating that Empowerment. Visualize this red ball growing brighter, breathing into it; as you do so, imagine that you're feeling centered in your power, will, and self-determination.

Step 4: Visualize both of these red spheres of light, at your tailbone and below your navel, growing brighter and their emanation growing larger. Eventually see the two merging together and creating rays of light that fill your body. These rays of light emanate out your skin and create a shell of red light upon the surface of your skin all the way around you—your Second Skin. Trace this from your head down to your toes, over the front of your face, the back of your head, your ears, your neck, your shoulders, your whole torso front and back, your hips and pelvis, your buttocks, into your legs, down your knees, your shins, your calves, your feet. Every square inch of you is covered on every side by this layer of strong red light, and it is fueled by your navel and root chakras.

Step 5: Take a couple of minutes to feel this layer of strength and protection. Say your affirmations and feel their power:

I am protected.

I am strong and resilient.

My energy is my own.

I assert my right to boundaries.

I am centered in my truth and power.

Step 6: Take your mental snapshot.

Step 7: Let go of the visual in your navel and root. Imagine that this Second Skin is now fully built around you; it is a permanent shield that will stay there without your visualization or awareness to fuel it.

Step 8: Open your eyes and walk out into your world.

When You Are Blocked

As explained in the Third Eye Empowerment chapter, we experience more than just the physical sensations that our physical senses bring us as we move through the world. In addition to the sights, sounds, smells, tastes, and textures we encounter through our physical body, on the level of our energy body, we encounter vibrations from everyone and everything. When we walk around without affirming any energetic filter or boundary, we absorb these energies and it may affect us physically, emotionally, mentally, or in any combination of these three.

There is a simple example I like to use to understand this: Imagine you are on a bus, sitting next to someone who, unbeknownst to you, is very angry. You are minding your own business, reading your newspaper or checking your phone, but sitting next to the angry person for some time. When you get off the bus, you have shifted for the worse in some way:

- If you're someone prone to taking in energy physically, perhaps you now have a headache or a stomachache; you start reviewing what you've eaten to understand why.

- If you're someone who tends to take things on emotionally, you may suddenly find yourself irritated and would find some outlet for that irritation. Perhaps you become irritated at the person in front of you who is walking slowly, whereas on another day that wouldn't bother you.

- If you're someone who takes energies on mentally, the content of your thoughts may change. While contemplating an interaction with your boss, you may suddenly find your thoughts becoming angrier though initially you were not angry.

In all three cases, you've taken on the energy of someone else's anger, and it's now manifested as your own, physically, emotionally, or mentally. We do this all the time. We are even more prone to absorb energies from those with whom we are in close relationships, something we will get into more in the next chapter. We are all part of an energy matrix, and to some extent it is natural and normal that there are constant energetic exchanges between us. But part of the process of working with your energy body is learning to stand in your own energetic integrity, and this is really what the Second Skin is about.

Most of the ways in which we absorb others' energies are not so straightforward. We're simply going about our day, and experiencing a constantly changing river of physical, emotional, and mental states, and have very little awareness of the true cause of these shifts. Usually we think it's due to something that has happened *to* us. We think we have a stomachache because of that heavy bagel we just ate, that we're annoyed because the woman in front of us is walking slowly, that we're angry at our boss because he did something wrong. But in fact, on another day, if we'd sat next to a cheerful person, none of this would have affected us in the same way, and we'd never know the difference.

For most of us, this unconscious absorbency is our default mode, and your default mode may be even more compromised by your own personal conditioning or empathic tendencies. The Second Skin can help you to shift your entire way of being in the world, and, ultimately, it can be part of your shift from *consumer* of energies to *creator* of energies. Instead of your energetic state being a product of the people and forces you come into contact with, you can have the energetic integrity to control your own energy, and positively impact the people and places you are around.

Using the Second Skin

Most of us are bombarded by stimuli all day—sensory and energetic—at a level and pace beyond anything prior generations have experienced, making it extremely difficult for us to maintain our energetic integrity. The Second Skin can help us to do so, but as with the development of most positive habits, it takes time. Research indicates habits take at least six weeks to solidify, and that's the estimate I like to use with the Second Skin. You may feel the shift happen faster or slower; overall, I recommend doing the full activation every day in the morning for six weeks, reactivating quickly throughout your day as needed. You can of course use the Second Skin more ad hoc than this, but if you believe you have issues with absorbing others' energy, consider taking this time to develop it as a new default way of carrying your energy.

Here are some specific examples of when you may want to consciously reactivate your Second Skin during your day when you are in this habit-forming period, or if you are using the Second Skin on a more as-needed basis:

- Before heading into a crowd—mass transit, traffic, a concert, a mall.
- Before interacting with anyone you know normally impacts you negatively.
- Before interacting with someone with whom you have difficulty enforcing boundaries of any type—e.g., you have difficulty saying no, stating your opinion, or voicing your preference. Perhaps combine with the Throat Matrix.

- Before any situation you find draining. Perhaps combine with the Navel Fire.

- Before any encounter in which you really need to stand your ground.

- Whenever you feel that your thoughts are jumping erratically, or your emotions are swinging.

- After you realize you're feeling drained from any of the above. Perhaps combine with the Sacral Lotus or Navel Fire, depending on what kind of energy you most need a boost from to recover.

- Whenever you notice your physical, emotional, or mental state has shifted for the worse and there is not an obvious trigger.

- In the days leading up to and during your menstrual period. (More on this in the Women's Energetics section.)

There are also specific life phases and transitions during which it may be helpful to work with the Second Skin more intensely. Here are some examples:

- When attempting to let go of comfort eating or using excess weight as an artificial boundary (as in Toni's story earlier) as part of a comprehensive diet and exercise transformation.

- During a phase in which you are the focus of others' attention to a greater degree than in the past. For example, you are teaching a class for the first time, giving presentations or lectures, or involved in large meetings or workshops.

- When you have just moved to a location with a higher population density than where you've lived in the past or are in crowds more often (for example, a change in commute that requires more time in mass transit or traffic).

- During the early stage of pregnancy (more on that in the next section).

- During perimenopause (more on this too!).

When it comes to using the Second Skin in order to improve your boundaries, you may need to take a deeper look at some of the conditioning we have discussed and how it's contributing to your lack of boundaries. Do you feel responsible for others' emotions? Do you feel unworthy and want to be needed? Are you people-pleasing? If so, why? Do you feel you don't have a right to assert boundaries or what you want? Depending on your answer, working with some of the other Chakra Empowerments in tandem with the Second Skin may benefit you.

Also helpful is developing your self-awareness around physical, emotional, and mental shifts, and questioning them from an energetic perspective. One of the most important questions you can ask yourself regarding this awareness is *Is this mine?* When you suspect it's not, let it go as quickly as you can. In terms of the example used above, imagine you got off that bus, noticed the shift right away, and said, "Wait a minute, I wasn't feeling (or thinking) this a second ago, why am I now? What just shifted? Is this mine?"

Women's Energetics: Your Energetic Cycles and Phases

In addition to the conditioning factors that often inhibit women's ability and sense of our right to enforce boundaries, there are also contributing energetic technical factors. We are beings of nature and as such have cycles and phases. Our cycles and phases correspond to our reproductive life, and our energy body shifts along with the corresponding physical changes. Many contemporary women are energetically disconnected from menstruation, fertility phases, pregnancy, perimenopause, and menopause, approaching them as medical, and therefore purely physical, events. But reconnecting to the ebb and flow of our energetic receptivity allows us to work with our power in a very beneficial way.

As we've already covered, our energy bodies are more naturally open and inward-pulling than men's. The sacral chakra is centripetal and receptive; because our energy is seated here, our entire energy body is as well. However, the intensity of this centripetal force ebbs and flows along with our hormonal shifts and reproductive cycles. Our chakras are in fact intricately connected to our endocrine system, and each chakra also corresponds to different organs and glands in our body. Our sacral chakra, the seat of our energy body, is linked to our ovaries and all our reproductive organs, so this physical system and our sacral chakra move in synchronicity with each other.

This ebb and flow relationship occurs between more solid and more emanating energy bodies—and the relationship is a very open and receptive one. We feel the difference in terms of our energetic sensitivity. When our energy body is more solid, it is less energetically sensitive and less prone to taking in energies from the outside. It is closer to having our Second Skin activated on its own. When our energy body is in its more open state, we are extremely sensitive to energy we come into contact with. We are constantly moving between these two states—our maximum level of solidity and our maximum level of sensitivity in accordance with our hormonal cycles and phases, like the waxing and waning of the moon.

One way to visualize this shifting is to think of the Sacral Lotus itself opening and closing. If you have ever seen a lotus in person, it is actually quite a hardy and sturdy flower. When we are at our maximum state of solidity, our lotus also has this hardy and sturdy quality. It is open and emanating its full power; in the face of that, other energies are burned off and not absorbed. When we are at our most sensitive, this flower closes into a blossom as if in self-protection, and the power turns inward. It is not gone; instead, it is in a gathering and regenerating stage, and therefore more vulnerable to outside energies entering. Of course, this is when our Second Skin is the most useful—it is like the sacral chakra's two surrounding, or "big brother," chakras, the root and navel, are providing protection.

Other factors contribute to our energetic ebb and flow besides our reproductive cycles and phases. Though not all women experience these cycles with the same level of intensity, here is a general overview:

- *Menstrual Cycle:* Our energy body is at its most solid and emanating at the peak of our fertility when we are ovulating, and at its most open and sensitive when we are menstruating. In between we are shifting between the two. The transition is not usually evenly spaced, however—it starts slowly and picks up quickly in the days just before we ovulate or begin menstruating. Therefore, the days just before ovulation and just before menstruation (corresponding to PMS) are when the changes are most tumultuous. In the case of ovulating, we are solidifying quickly during these days, and in the case of the days before our period, we are rapidly becoming more sensitive.

- *Fertile Years:* Our most fertile years are, on average, from ages sixteen to thirty-five, when our menstrual cycle is typically the most intense and regular. This energy cycle is also the most pronounced, and the swings between the two maximum states is the most prominent. In other words, our energy body is fluctuating a lot of the time, in a constant dance between these two states.

• *Pregnancy:* In the first trimester of pregnancy, we are often in our most sensitive state, similar to menstruation, as our body adjusts to the lack of a cycle and our sacral chakra begins to channel more energy into our womb. In the same way, our body reprioritizes sending nutrients first to our placenta and then to the rest of our body. Our sacral chakra directs more energy to our womb, so the rest of our energy body is not solid and emanating during this time. However, as our pregnancy adjusts, our sacral chakra actually opens. It is the spiritual and energetic portal for birth, mirroring the physical portal our body provides. As it opens in preparation for this, our sacral emanates more and more energy, and we are actually in quite a solid state energetically—others may perceive this as our pregnancy glow.

• *Perimenopause:* Perimenopause is the transition phase before menopause, before our cycle stops entirely. It may last anywhere from a few months to several years. Most women experience it to some degree during their forties. Our cycles become irregular, and we begin to experience the classic physical symptoms of menopause off and on. Energetically, our energy body also tends to become erratic, along with our periods; for some women, this is the first time that our physical and energetic bodies are not in sync. Our physical cycles and our energy cycles become separated from one another. As a result, we may experience periods of intense sensitivity, or intense energetic strength seemingly randomly, and it doesn't feel within our control. There is actually a lot of potential to work with this shift for greater growth, but from a boundary perspective, we can be left feeling unprotected.

• *Menopause:* After menopause, we stabilize into a new normal in which our energy swings are much less dramatic. We still do experience an ebb and flow in our energy body, but the shifts are not as distinct. If we process this well, it can be extremely liberating—for the first time, our level of openness or solidity can be within our control. This is also possible premenopause but is harder to do—prior to menopause, it is usually more helpful to adapt our activities to where we are in our cycle or phase. Postmenopause, we can own the power fully to control the opening and closing of our sacral chakra at any time.

The relevance of understanding these cycles in terms of the Second Skin is to recognize that in your more sensitive phases when your sacral chakra is in its most inward-turning phase, you are in the most need of the Second Skin. At these times, your root and navel chakras on either side of your sacral play a particularly important shielding role.

Part of your personal work may be releasing any aversion you have to the very idea that your energy body waxes and wanes along with your reproductive phases and cycles. I find some contemporary women resist this because it feels as if we are being reduced to our reproductive function. We aren't; recognizing and honoring these cycles enables you to maximize your power, not diminish it. Men have energetic cycles too; they are just less pronounced. Because ours are more pronounced, we can *use* them with awareness.

We are at our most intuitive and insightful during our sensitive and inward-pulling phases, and at our most productive and charismatic during our outward and solid phases. To the extent that you can make use of these phases along these lines, it can be tremendously effective. Of course, you can't reorganize your entire life in this way, but you don't need to. Simply attempting to give yourself some space and time to contemplate during your sensitive phases and really going for what you want during your solid phases will yield tangible results. Awareness is power.

I'm sometimes asked how birth control pills, implants, and related methods affect these energetic cycles and phases. The short answer is that they blunt the energetic phasing. There is still an ebb and a flow, but it is much less pronounced. Some women find this helpful—after all, it is easier to learn to work with these cycles when they are less intense. And if your life doesn't allow you a lot of room to adapt your life to your cycle, you may find it easier. However, some women find this energetic blunting limiting, as they feel out of touch with their full intuition. Obviously, this shouldn't be the primary reason you go on or off any particular birth control method—your procreative choices and sexual activity should be driving that. This information is offered in the spirit of helpfulness and may influence what method is right for you at different times in your life. It is information for you to consider—just like awareness is power, information is power.

Patricia was normally very grounded and centered in her power but needed help—she felt as though she had hit her limit with several stressors all occurring at once in her life. A successful graphic designer, she had recently been promoted to a management position within her firm, which involved spending a lot more time in meetings and presenting to clients than she was used to. She felt these duties made her frazzled and unfocused; she left every meeting with her mind buzzing and missed her solitary time alone in front of her computer working through ideas.

At home, Patricia had a husband and two busy teenage children. Her husband had begun traveling more for his own job, leaving Patricia with more of the kid shuttling. She didn't mind this but found she was having a hard time handling the increased contact with other moms while waiting for her kids to get out of their respective sports practices. Her eldest was a high school junior, and it seemed all any of these moms wanted to talk about was the college application process, and where their kids were applying. While normally not one to stress about such things, Patricia often found herself feeling anxiety after these encounters—was she doing enough to help her own daughter? Did she need SAT tutoring? When would they possibly find time to visit colleges? What if they couldn't afford the one her daughter wanted?

The biggest stressor in Patricia's life was her aging mother. Her father had passed away three years before, and in the years since, her mother had experienced one health problem after another. She was now in a rehabilitation home after hip surgery, and her caretakers had told Patricia they did not think her mother could return to living alone. They urged her to find an assisted living facility, something her mother adamantly refused. There were financial constraints to this as well, as it didn't look like either her mother's savings or insurance would cover the cost. Patricia tried to visit her mother every other day, but frequently left upset as her mother cycled through anger, bitterness, and sadness.

On top of all of this, Patricia was exhibiting the first signs of perimenopause and not sleeping well. She would frequently awake and cycle through all of her worries—the big client presentation at work the next day, her daughter's college application process, her tight carpool schedule, financial worries, her mother's care. She swung wildly during these nighttime vigils between anxiety, hopelessness, frustration, and fear. She knew these were all problems that had solutions, and though she was normally quite rational about working through things like this, she could not seem to access that side of herself right now. During her day, too, she felt she was on an emotional roller coaster, uncharacteristically swinging wildly through moods. She wondered if she needed hormonal therapy for this but really did not want to pursue it due to other health risk factors.

I had known Patricia for some time and had seen her handle some incredibly stressful experiences in her life, so I knew her current struggles were unusual for her. We talked more about her perimenopausal symptoms, and I explained how a woman's subtle body can swing erratically during this time and that she may be absorbing other people's energies more so than in the past. She was taking in the demanding energies of clients in meetings, the anxiety of other moms, and the anger and depression of her own mother, and it was too much for her energy body. The mood swings were not entirely hormonal but energetic, as she took on the emotions of all these other people in her life.

We decided she would work intensively with the Second Skin for a few weeks before making any medication decisions. The plan was for her to activate the Second Skin for ten to fifteen minutes every day before leaving her home. We added an affirmation about stabilizing her energy body and emotions. She then did the Second Skin before meetings, contact with other moms, and visiting her own mom. Within a week, Patricia reported feeling more stable and less stressed and that her mental clarity was beginning to return. At this point, we added some third eye work to help her improve her ability to intuit when energies were affecting her, so she could consciously use them for intuitive purposes—and halt herself from absorbing them. She did some inner personal work related to the heart chakra and the feeling that she could not ask for help, and she began to talk more openly with her husband about the support she needed.

With all this work and her continued use of the Second Skin, Patricia felt like she began carrying herself differently. She experienced the sense of shielding her energy body without effort most of the time, filtering what she took in. As she reclaimed her energetic integrity, she also began to feel more like her old self, able to calmly assess what needed to be done. Her promotion and life stressors no longer felt like too much for her, and she was able to meet her challenges. She was able to sleep again and decided to continue through perimenopause without hormonal treatment for the time being.

Whether it's PMS, early pregnancy, or perimenopause, during our most sensitive energetic periods we are more prone to take in energy from others, and the result may be erratic emotions. Although of course hormones may play a role—and I would never discourage anyone from seeing a doctor and talking it through—often using the Second Skin to stabilize your energy field will help and may even be enough on its own. Interestingly, many women who had irregular cycles even preperimenopause have told me that working with the Second Skin helped to stabilize their cycle—the connections between our energy body, emotions, and physical body run deep, and changes we make on any one level often cascade to the others.

Sexual Trauma Healing: Your Right to Boundaries

If you are a sexual trauma survivor, working with the Second Skin can benefit you in a very essential way: helping you reclaim and affirm on every level your right and ability to enforce boundaries: physical, emotional, energetic, and any other sort. Sexual trauma is a violation of our most personal boundary. If yours occurred when you were a child—and especially if it was by an adult you trusted, you may have internalized the idea that you don't have the *right* to enforce boundaries. If it occurred later in your life, your faith in your *ability* to do so may have been shaken. Working with the Second Skin regularly is a way of affirming over and over, to every level of your psyche, "I control the energies of all types that enter my being," and "I have a right to assert this control."

You may also have an increased sense of vulnerability stemming from your trauma. As I discussed in the root chakra chapter, empowering the root energies of safety and resilience is very important for strengthening your energetic foundation, and the Second Skin can be an additional Empowerment for this. However, your heightened sense of vulnerability may cause you to be especially prone to relating to the Second Skin solely as a protective shield, such that you would fall into the habit of judging all energies and situations as only "good" or "bad." Remember that what you are really trying to empower is your ability to control how energies affect you; you are not seeking to control your environment or avoid all negativity in the attempt to feel safe. When you truly own your Second Skin abilities, the possibilities for your life are opened, not further limited, because you trust in your capacity to handle whatever you encounter.

Sexual trauma survivors often also have a harder time relating to their reproductive cycles and phases in a positive way, due to disassociating from the body or from physical experiences linked to being female. We talked about this in the context of body image in the Sacral Lotus chapter, but it's often also relevant as it relates to menstruation, fertility cycles, pregnancy, perimenopause, and menopause. It's worth thinking about your attitude toward these natural cycles of your body. Do you welcome them as part of your feminine power? Do you view them solely as a hindrance or (even worse) as "dirty"? Are you able to speak openly with your doctor or sexual partners about things going on physically for you related to these cycles?

Blocks to doing so affect many women, not only sexual trauma survivors, because of historical views on menstruation as unclean and taboos on speaking about female sexuality. In an age where Viagra ads are everywhere, the avoidance and silencing seem particularly ridiculous, although they illustrate well another way in which feminine energy and all things linked to it are still suppressed. Work on becoming more comfortable with these aspects of yourself and on healing latent feelings of shame about them with the Sacral Lotus. Experiment too with using the Second Skin in relation to your cycles and owning the power you can feel through synchronizing your energy work with these cycles.

NINE
Web of Light:
Your Relationships

Related Chakras: Your entire energy body

Energies: Energetic exchange in relationships
with other people in your life

Use For: Cutting lines with individuals with whom you need to
cease or lessen energetic interaction, clearing lines with those with
whom you have a supportive relationship but a dysfunction has
developed, activating the ability to open and close supportive lines

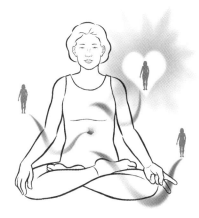

We are each part of a web of energy. To imagine your web, take a moment to visualize—or even draw if you like—the following:

- Picture yourself in the center of a series of three concentric circles.
- In the circle closest to you sit all the people you are closest to in your life—immediate family members and closest friends. Imagine there are lines of pure light connecting you to each of these people, connecting them if they have relationships with each other.
- In the next circle beyond them, picture those people with whom you regularly interact but do not have a deep emotional or psychological relationship with—coworkers, neighbors, acquaintances, your doctor, your children's teachers, etcetera. Now imagine lines extending from you to each of them. There may also be lines between some of these people or between people in your inner circle and people in this circle. Don't worry about imagining all these lines; generally visualize lines intersecting between and within circles.
- Now visualize a third circle further out from you that contains people in your larger world that you may see once in a while but don't interact regularly with. This might be clerks at the grocery store, the librarian at the library, distant relatives, old friends with whom you don't interact with much, or friends of friends. You won't be able to bring to mind all of these people, but bring to mind enough of them that you can create a robust circle. Imagine lines of light extending from you to these people as well. Now generally imagine all of the lines that might exist between these people and people in your inner two circles.
- Beyond this, imagine all the people in the rest of the world. Although you may not have energy lines to any more people beyond your third circle, the people in your three circles do. Imagine lines of light reaching out from each of them into their own webs of light.

It gets complicated quickly, doesn't it? While you probably don't have active energy lines with all of these people you have imagined, you do interact with all of them to some extent, which means there is some amount of energy effect. There are a lot of different models for thinking about our relationships energetically, and in our last chapter, Second Skin, we focused on in-person energetic exchanges. However, we exchange energy within our entire web of relationships, and they can affect us even when we are not in an individual's presence. The energy of someone in our web—particularly someone in our inner circle—may affect us even when we are not with them. Thinking in terms of energy lines will help us visualize these kinds of energy exchanges.

In the sense in which we will explore them here, energy lines are not the same as energy cords, contracts, or other terms you may have heard. Energy lines are involved in cords and contracts (and working with Web of Light will certainly help with those energy issues), but they are not the focus of this Empowerment. The Web of Light is an everyday Empowerment tool meant to help you consciously manage your energy within your web on an ongoing basis.

Specifically, you will use the Web of Light to cut energy lines with people from your past who are no longer in your life, or with whom you feel your dynamic has become dysfunctional. There may also be people in your life with whom you have an ongoing relationship (and/or you care very much about), but an energetic problem has developed. You will clear these energy lines. After that, you will empower the lines with people who love and support you and activate your ability to open and close all lines—yes, even these—because energy exchange should be your choice.

What does it mean to have a dysfunctional energy line? Generally speaking, energy flows both ways; put simply, a line is therefore problematic for you if interacting with the person negatively affects you or you sense their moods or issues are affecting you negatively, even when you don't interact. For example, say your best friend is going through a difficult divorce, and you want to support her but feel as though you are getting pulled down emotionally with her. You feel stressed and sad even when you are not speaking with her, yet there is nothing in your own life to trigger these feelings. The Second Skin will help when you speak with her, but you are very likely absorbing some of her energy even when you are not interacting because of your ongoing relationship. In this case, clearing this line with the Web of Light will help you to redefine the relationship's energy dynamics.

The level to which someone else can affect you through an energy line is directly proportional to the intimacy of your relationship with them. So, a friend you see almost every day may have as much of an effect as your brother with whom you have a strong history and family line but don't see very often. In general, whomever forms a big part of our history, family, or shared time are going to be the individuals whose energy affects us the most.

Amongst energy lines, the most prominent types are these:

- **Family.** Within this category of lines, parent-child lines are unique; we will talk about mother-child lines in the Women's Energetics section.

- **Ongoing Sexual Relationships.** Sex between individuals, regardless of gender, creates a very specific type of energy line. The most intense line is of course with our current spouse or lover, but we may also have old energetic lines to individuals from past sexual and romantic relationships.

- **Other Relationship-Based Lines.** All of our other lines with friends and acquaintances, the intensity of which is based on the length of our relationship, our level of emotional intimacy, and the frequency of our interaction.

When we interact with someone with whom we have a strong line, it will affect us more strongly than an interaction with someone whom we have just met. If you interact in person with a stranger who is angry, you may pick up that anger, as in the example from the Second Skin chapter. But if you interact with your mother over the phone and she is angry—even if it is not directed at you—that is likely to have a stronger impact on you, and you are likely to take on some of her anger, and in turn be affected physically, emotionally, or mentally, in much the same way as the "stranger on the bus" example of the previous chapter.

In some ways, thinking in terms of energy lines is a cold and technical way of discussing relationships. After all, humans are intrinsically social; energy exchange is normal and natural. There is a lot more to consider than whether a particular person drains or energizes you—feelings and history matter, and compassion is always the best choice. Working with the Web of Light is *not* about cutting certain people out of your life or limiting interactions with others. It may not be about externally changing your relationships at all. It is about empowering you with awareness and choice within the dynamic of the relationships you currently have.

With this Empowerment, we have moved to another level of working energetically. The Web of Light is not chakra specific, and the remaining Empowerments involve many parts of your energy body. For that reason, it's not relevant to talk in terms of specific chakra blocks or memories of when you may have felt these energies before. Those sections won't appear in the remaining chapters; instead, we will focus a lot more on Women's Energetics.

Suki wanted help managing the stress and insomnia she was experiencing related to problems members of her family were facing. Her husband was working on a make-or-break work project resulting in long hours and consistent stress. Her ten-year-old son's best friend had recently moved away, so her son was lonely and unhappy at school. Suki's mother had recently moved to an independent living facility but now feared it was a mistake and was second-guessing her decision.

Suki was uncharacteristically thrown off balance by all their unhappiness and stress. She recognized that none of these issues were life-threatening, and she was doing her best to support each person: helping her husband proofread his writing, arranging playdates for her son, and talking through options with her mother. But she found herself high-strung all day and unable to sleep at night, spinning in her mind over potentials she could not control—what if her husband's computer crashed? What if her son had no one to play with at recess? Would the independent living facility sue her mother for breach of contract? Then her mind would spin to other worries: Had she turned off the stove? Answered that email? Did the dog seem lethargic? Maybe he had cancer! Oh no, her son would really be devastated if something happened to him.

On and on it would go, and Suki had never experienced anything like it. She considered herself a generally calm and pragmatic person. For this reason, I decided we would start with Web of Light, as I suspected that Suki was taking on stress and anxiety from each member of her family through her energy lines. Having three people in her inner energetic circle all going through a stressful time in their lives simultaneously had overwhelmed her energetically.

We focused first on her husband, then on her son, and finally on her mother, clearing the energy lines with each of them. We then activated Suki's ability to open and close these energy lines at will. We then did the Root Bowl to quell her anxiety. I asked Suki to repeat both exercises daily in the morning, and the Root Bowl again at night before bed.

In our next session, Suki reported there had been a definite improvement, and she was sleeping much better. Each morning after doing the Web of Light, she felt tremendously calm and centered. She used that as her touchstone throughout the day, and whenever she felt she was starting to worry too much about one or more of her family members, she quickly recleared the line and activated the Root Bowl through her snapshot memory. Doing this for a week had triggered her to think more deeply about how she viewed her role in her family as well as how she managed her energy with other people in her life. She embarked upon some longer-term personal work to heal some heart wounds causing her to feel overly responsible for her family's happiness at times, and to make use of the Second Skin to help her maintain her energetic integrity with everyone she encountered throughout her day.

It is important to recognize that in Suki's case, clearing the energy lines with her family members did not mean she supported them any less. On the contrary, she was able to support them more effectively because she was not so fatigued herself. Shifting our energy lines is about self-care, not cutting people off or heartlessness.

Activation Steps

Unlike the other Empowerments we have worked with so far, there is no specific chakra visual involved with Web of Light or memories of when you have experienced this energy before. However, there is some prep work you will need to do. The first time you use Web of Light, I suggest you sit down and identify three people: one person in your life with whom you would like to cut your energy line, one person with whom you would like to clear your energy line, and a third person with whom you would like to empower and gain more control over a line. Let's look at some examples of whom you might put in each category:

- *Cutting:* A past friend or lover with whom you no longer associate; someone who is still in your life but you feel you should not have an energy line with; someone from your past you are thinking about too much; someone you need to break ties with.

- *Clearing:* Someone from your valued inner circle but with whom a dysfunctional energetic dynamic has developed—perhaps there are lingering feelings of anger or resentment from a past conflict or other events and you would like an energetic reboot.

- *Empower and Activate:* Someone who supports you—a loving family member, mentor, teacher, or person you admire.

With these three people in mind, you can begin the Web of Light:

Step 1: As always, sit with your spine as straight as possible. Breathe into your body.

Step 2: Visualize the first person, the person with whom you would like to cut the line. Visualize them in a sphere of energy in front of you. Visualize a line of light from your navel center to theirs.

Step 3: Imagine your fingers as a pair of scissors and cut the line between yourself and them—just snip it. Imagine their end of the line is now going back into their body. Your end of the line is coming back into yours. Repeat up to three times if you feel you need to.

Step 4: Imagine that the person with whom you're cutting the line dissolves into light and fades away. Then take a few deep breaths focused on your own navel chakra, really centering in your own body.

Step 5: Now we will move on to the person with whom you would like to clear a line. Visualize this person in a sphere of light in front of you. Visualize a line of light from your heart chakra to theirs.

Step 6: In the center of this line between you, at the midpoint, visualize a bright golden dot of light. See this golden dot spreading out toward both of you so it elongates as it reaches toward both of your hearts. As it does so, imagine that any negative emotions or dysfunction is releasing off of the line as dark debris. See this golden light spread until the entire line, from your heart to theirs, is clear with gold light.

Step 7: Now imagine a tiny doorway close to your own heart, near where the line comes into your heart. Hold your hand in front of your heart chakra (or wherever you are visualizing this line) and swing your hand back and forth like a door, imagining opening and closing the line. After visualizing this a few times, leave the door closed for now. Imagine the person on the other end dissolving into light.

Step 8: Now we will work with someone you want to empower your line with. Visualize this person in front of you and imagine an energy line in your solar plexus, just below your rib cage between your navel and heart chakras, with a line going into their solar plexus.

Step 9: As you did at the end of the line clearing process, visualize a door on this line, close to your own body. Visualize this door opening and see the entire energy line lighting up with beautiful golden light. See this vibrant gold light flowing back and forth across this line.

Step 10: Holding your hand where you imagine this door, now visualize yourself opening and closing the line as you mirror this action with the movements of your hand. Leave the door open for now but still imagine the person and their line dissolves for the time being.

Step 11: Let all the visuals and thoughts of all three people go. Sit centered in your energy body, and say the affirmations:

I cut energy lines with people who are not healthy for me.
I cleanse energy lines with people I care about but with whom a problematic energy dynamic has developed.
I empower energy lines with people who support and nurture me.
I stand in my own energetic integrity and power.
I decide with whom and when I share or exchange energy.

Step 12: You can end here, or you can end by activating another Empowerment. For example, if you were cutting a line with someone for whom it was difficult to do, activate the Navel Fire. If you were clearing a line that caused you anxiety or upset, activate the Root Bowl. If you were empowering a line with someone you love, you may want to activate the Heart Star.

Do not get too caught up in where exactly the energy lines are in each case. For this kind of energy line work, it is fine to use the navel, heart, and solar plexus locations given in this example. In reality, we have multiple entrance points for energy into our body with most people in our lives, and it is not necessary to locate each of these. As with all the Empowerments, the visual is activating an energetic shift and psychological process, and to do this it does not need to be literal.

Using the Web of Light

The Web of Light is an energetic tool that empowers your ability to affirm and take control of your energetic exchanges, but just like with the Second Skin, it can become problematic if you get into a mode of thinking you'll just cut lines with someone as soon as you feel negativity from them and empower lines with people you want something from. We have different kinds of exchanges with the people in our life; you can have a negative exchange with someone you love deeply or a positive exchange with a stranger on the street. Life is beautifully messy that way, and this Empowerment won't help you if it turns you into an energetic control freak.

On a daily basis, Web of Light is best employed when there's an issue, and you should keep it simple. If there's someone from your past you need to let go of, cut the line. If there's someone you care about but a problematic dynamic has developed between you two, clear the line. When there is someone with whom you feel you need to take more conscious control of how you interact and/or would like to empower further positive interactions, affirm the line and work with the door. Of course, you do not need to do all three types of line work every time you do the Web of Light. Although at first it may be helpful to do so in a controlled environment at home (as with all the Empowerments), most of the instances in which you use this Empowerment in your day will be quick and focused on just one type of line.

For example, if someone from your past is on your mind a lot but you don't want to make contact, you can cut the line quickly every time you think of them. Examples are former romantic partners or friends or family you've had to distance yourself from and don't wish to reengage with. Of course, there may be other personal work you need to do to heal any lingering emotional wounds or doubts from this past relationship, and other Chakra Empowerments may assist. In the moment of thinking about the person, cut the line and move on.

An example of a good everyday use of line clearing is when you've just had a negative exchange with someone you care about. Perhaps you've just had an argument with your daughter and you want to clear out the energy before you walk back into the room to try to talk to her again. You also want to make sure you don't get triggered into anger by her agitated state. You could do the line clearing work, and imagine you are closing the energy door. You might also want to activate the Heart Star to help you enter the room with compassion or the Root Bowl to calm any anxiety.

Closing an energy line does not prevent you from meeting the world with compassion. Most of the time when you choose to close the door on a line, it is to affirm you will not *take any energy in* from that person. You may want to do this when you are comforting someone so that you can truly emanate from your heart the compassion and nurturing you would like to give them without taking in their own sadness or fear. Working with the Web of Light is also not a substitute for actually communicating with people in your life. If there is a bad dynamic that has developed between you and a loved one, you need to talk it through, in which case the Web of Light may help support you in the conversation.

Although Web of Light will mostly be of use to you in these daily kinds of situations, working with it regularly for a longer term period can transform your relationships. One way to do this is to work your way through line work with all of the inner circle people in your life, and perhaps a few second circle people. Sit down one day and make a list of all your different relationships and the different categories that they fall into: family, friends, spouse or significant other, children, coworkers, neighbors, other associations. Then for each one, write down how you would like to work with that energy. Would you like to cut, cleanse, or open/close that line? Then work your way through these over a period of time, two or three per day.

This is a transformative and empowering process because it triggers introspection about your relationships. It forces you to contemplate how you are relating to the people in your life and how you are affecting each other. It also prompts you to own the ways you may be holding on to the past and helps you let go. It will help you identify conversations you may need to have in order to change or even save certain relationships. In the busyness of our lives, it is easy to let things go; relationships can deteriorate slowly without our noticing. Working with Web of Light regularly can help you to take responsibility for the quality of your relationships.

Women's Energetics: Mother-Child Lines and Sexual Lines

Two types of energy lines are particularly relevant for women—sexual lines and mother-child lines. Both are lines that affect our sacral chakras and therefore have a disproportionate impact on our overall well-being and personal power because the sacral is the seat of our energy body. Both can also be complicated to talk about; doing so can sound like justification for two outdated sexist views: that women should limit their sexual partners while men don't need to, and that women should bear the brunt of child-rearing. As should be clear by now, I don't support either of these views. My reason for sharing this information is that it can empower women by helping us to understand our energy body dynamics and influence our energetic self-care.

Sex is a very unique kind of energy exchange and one of the most powerful. It can, after all, create life. But even when it does not do that, it is an energetic meeting between individuals that cannot happen any other way. Its power is such that virtually every religious and spiritual tradition has something to say about it. On one end we have religions that limit sex to procreative purposes or place strict moral limits upon it. On the other end are spiritual traditions that incorporate sacred sexuality, some of which even uphold that sex is the highest spiritual experience we can have.

The latter view is based on the ways that our chakras can open and connect with each other, particularly the chakras of the feminine pathway—the sacral, heart, and third eye. As we've already discussed, our sacral chakra pulls energy inward and is linked to our procreative function. It is like fertile ground energetically, waiting to be planted in ... and what gets planted far more often than conception is *sexual energy lines.*

Women are energetically prone to developing lines with their sexual partners, something that applies regardless of whether you are gay, straight, or bi. While it's possible to have sex without a line forming, it very often does. This is in addition to whatever other lines form based on the emotions of a relationship. If you are in a long-term relationship, you will likely have heart lines and power (navel) lines form as well, and perhaps others. Because our sacral chakra is naturally inward-pulling, these lines are often more of a problem for us than for men because we bring energy in on these lines from our sexual partners—potentially to include past and present partners. And because our sacral chakra is the natural seat of our energy body, this energy can weigh us down. In other words, our energy body, and, by extension, our state of awareness, may be subtly impacted by the emotions and state of our current and past lovers.

This is not the case for all women, and the effect is normally subtle. If your sexual relationships have been with other women, the impact is harder to discern. But if you feel at all like there is some part of you holding on to past relationships—if, for example, you think of past lovers frequently—and/or if you feel as if your emotions are very erratic and you cannot find a reason in your day-to-day life, then going through a period of extensive line cutting with all of your past sexual partners may be very helpful to you. It will help you to clear out your sacral chakra of any lingering lines. It also may help you reclaim any lost energy from those encounters—any energy you gave out in a relationship and haven't taken back as your own.

Like sensitivity, sexual sacral lines have an upside. In a committed, healthy relationship, our sacral line with our partner is part of what makes sacred sexuality and sexual bliss possible for both partners. It also often forms the anchor for a positive, loving relationship—as the energetic fertile ground, roots can flourish in our sacral. This doesn't mean you should only have sex in a committed relationship, it just means bring awareness to what you are doing. If it's not a long-term relationship, cut the line.

Another kind of line that is specific to women's sacral chakras, and that also needs to be managed well, is the mother-child line. This is a particular line between a birth mother's sacral chakra and her children's navel chakras;

it mirrors the physical umbilical cord. If a birth mother raises her child, this energetic line extends throughout the mother's lifetime, although it changes over time, as the child becomes more independent. If a child is put up for adoption, this line will fade, and new lines are formed with adoptive parents. All parents form energy lines with their children, and in fact much of what I will say about mother-child energy lines can be true of all parental lines. Fathers tend to form heart lines, not sacral lines, however, whereas mothers form both.

The main purpose of the mother-child energetic line is for the mother to support the baby as needed with her own energy; primarily, it is meant to be an outgoing line for the mother. We use this line naturally to send energy to our child when they are sick or upset. However, as the child grows, the amount the mother supports energetically in this way should lessen—her child should be gaining energetic independence along with his or her physical independence. Problems arise when a mother tries to hold on to or control her child through this line or doesn't let go when she should.

Although the growing energetic independence of the child happens gradually and is slightly different for each child—just like physical and psychological development—there are certain benchmarks. During the first three to six months, sometimes referred to as the "fourth trimester," the energetic connection between mother and child is particularly intense. The first major shift toward energetic independence happens around six months of age. Then another big shift happens at around eighteen months, and again at three years old. At six and twelve years old, additional big shifts happen; in fact, after twelve years, this particular line should be almost closed in terms of its initial supportive function.

By adulthood, there should be complete energetic independence. There still may be a strong line between mother and child, but it should now be based on the heart, not the sacral line. If we don't let go enough, our child never gains that energetic independence. On the other hand, if we don't acknowledge this energetic dependence when our child is young, they may not feel as if they're getting the energy they need from us. So, it's important to recognize this line and balance your own energetic needs with those of your child.

A lot of women in today's world feel overwhelmed by this line when they first have children, especially if they have children later (as I myself did) and have therefore gone a longer time in their life with their own energetic integrity. It's important to recognize this line will weaken over time and can be augmented by other people. Though it may feel this way at times, it does *not* mean you have to be with your children all the time and no one else can fulfill their needs. Some women feel this line so intensely that they end up cutting others out, even their partners, from helping with childcare or the energetic support of their children. You need to be very conscious of how this line works, ask for help, and, of course, engage in self-care.

Self-care is where the Web of Light comes in. You can and should clear lines with your children as needed and work with the door open-and-close Empowerment. You should be able to close this door when you are particularly drained or when your children are relying on you too much. Clearing lines doesn't prevent you from loving and nurturing them—that comes from your heart, not your sacral. There are also times you may want to empower and affirm the door's opening—for example, if your child is away from home for the first time and feeling nervous. And if you work with the Web of Light from the time your children are young, you will be attuned to it by the time they are in their tweens and the door is closing. Then it's time to let go on that level and allow your relationship to shift.

There are situations in which you may also want to work with the Web of Light in relationship to this energy line with your own mother. If you feel as if she has not let you go and is seeking to control you in some way that is not healthy, cutting this line may help. Of course, we develop other lines with our mother, and if you are in an ongoing relationship with her, you may need to clear lines too.

Marley was trying to turn her life around after a series of abusive relationships. Raised by a neglectful, alcoholic mother and largely absent father, Marley had turned to boys in her teens as a substitute for love. She learned young that she could use sex as a means to get boys' attention, and while she yearned for true affection to grow from sex, more often she was used for a time and then ignored. In her late teens, Marley finally got what she thought she wanted—a boyfriend. She moved in with him but quickly discovered he was physically abusive. She stuck it out with him for two years, finally leaving after a particularly bad assault. She then found a new, older boyfriend who she thought was different but also turned out to be physically abusive.

Fortunately for Marley, she sought help with a domestic violence center after leaving this second boyfriend and began to get some support there to change her life. When I met her, she had been in counseling for a year, had a job, and was starting night school. She felt ready to begin meeting men again but was terrified she would repeat the same pattern. Highly intuitive, Marley wanted energetic help in addition to her counseling support.

We started with supported, intensive Web of Light work. Marley made a list of all the sexual partners she could remember, going back to her first encounter at age fourteen. I walked her through cutting lines with the first three boys on her list, and then we did Root Bowl and Navel Fire work. I asked Marley to continue on her own through the rest of her list until the two longer term abusive relationships, which we would do together. I asked her to always do the Root Bowl and Navel Fire after, and to stop if the daily work was getting to be too much. I also told her to stop if any distressing memories were triggered through a particular line cutting.

To the contrary, Marley loved the daily work; she felt like she was taking back her past. She would often send healing to her young self through visualization, something she had been doing in counseling. A couple of the line cuttings had been emotional, as she remembered sexual encounters that had been assaults, though she had not recognized them as such at the time. However, she did not feel overwhelmed by these memories … only compassion for her young self.

Next, Marley and I together did longer line-cutting sessions on her two abusive boyfriends. She focused on sending them away, feeling they were completely in her past. She also felt she needed to cut the line with her mother, who was no longer in her life. After this, we began working with other Chakra Empowerments to support Marley's transformation, including building her a new support network and empowering her to envision a new life. Although she decided to hold off on seeing men again for some time, she continued with night school, made new friends, and began laying the groundwork for a new, healthier future.

Marley was able to do intensive line cutting work because she had a lot of support from me and her counselor. While some women can work in this way on their own, it's important not to overwhelm yourself. If you are cutting lines with people who abused you, you may need additional emotional support. Line cutting is not about recovering memories, but it sometimes happens; you'll want to be supported if it does. While I believe in our capacity to self-heal and think most of us have much more capability in this regard than we think, I also know that many of us can't do it alone. Honor your needs.

Sexual Trauma Healing: Taking Control of Your Energy

Energy line work through the Web of Light can be a very helpful part of healing from sexual abuse or assault. First of all, working with it in everyday situations can help you reclaim your sense of boundary (just as with the Second Skin) and strengthen your inner belief that you have a right to control the energies that come into your energy body. It is easy to say you believe this, but taking control with the use of these Empowerments will help bring your subtle body and unconscious into alignment with your affirmations.

If you were abused as a child, you may feel you need to cut lines with family members who did not protect or believe you and it is thus best for you to no longer see or talk to them. Whether your trauma was when you were a child or adult, there are likely others in your life who did not support you, and whom as part of your healing, you believe you need to remove from your life. If that is the case, cutting lines to affirm that may be helpful. Working to clear lines with individuals you are still interacting with but who do not yet seem able to understand what you have been through and support you may also be helpful. Neither are substitutes for communication, nor is there any guarantee it will help shift the dynamic between you. Even if nothing changes, know that it may help you feel more at peace with the state of the relationship and decrease the negative effect it has on you. Hopefully, you also have supportive people in your life who are helping you to heal; if that's the case, you may want to empower and affirm these lines.

We now come to the big questions that many sexual trauma survivors ask: "Do I still have an energy line to my abuser or assaulter?" "Could they still be affecting me?" "Do I need to cut this line?"

The answer varies. We cut energy lines indirectly all the time through other healing modalities; if you had a line, you may very well have cut it already through therapy or other healing you have done. It is not always necessary—or wise—to do so through an explicit Empowerment such as the Web of Light. For some survivors, doing so may be too traumatic—maybe you have worked very hard to stop thinking about your assaulter or abuser, and bringing up a visual of them in order to cut the line will only bring you backward in your healing, not forward. In this case, don't do it. If you have stopped thinking about your assaulter or abuser as often as you once did, you have already cut (or are in the process of cutting) the line through your other healing means. There is no reason to undertake this method.

On the other hand, many survivors do find this line cutting empowering. Most likely, you will need support if you choose to do so. You may want to undertake it in the company of a friend, counselor, or healer. Remember that this is not a memory exercise, and you do *not* need to even visualize your abuser or assaulter if you wish (in some cases, you may not know what they look like). You can visualize a dark shadow figure that represents their energy in your life. Then cut that line. Do it multiple times and see this figure disappear. They are gone from your life and your psyche. If you like, affirm this for yourself by saying, "I have no energetic line or connection with you. You do not affect me in any way. My life is my own."

This exercise can be a very powerful part of taking back your life and your power. Part of moving from "victim to survivor to thriver" (a popular #MeToo phrase) is getting to a place where your abuse or assault is simply part of your history. It has shaped you, but through your process of healing you no longer feel like it defines you or shadows you. This isn't something you can force, but as you work to heal, it will happen. Working with the Web of Light to let go of your past, and take control of your current energy, can be an important part of helping you get there.

TEN

Healing Rays:
Your Restorative Light

Related Chakras: Your sacral (second),
heart (fourth), and palm chakras

Energies: Healing, soothing, calming, regenerating,
releasing, dissolving, strengthening immunity

Use For: Speeding healing in your body, complementing other
healing modalities, including emotional healing

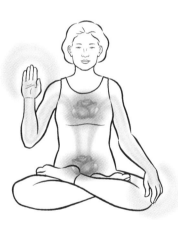

All healing is self-healing. Any medicines you take or procedures you undergo are meant to aid your own body in its return to health. If you take ibuprofen for a sprained ankle, it doesn't heal the damaged tissue; instead, it reduces the inflammation and limits your pain, which aids your body's ability to heal. If you take an antibiotic, it kills the bacteria that made you sick, but then your own body has to take over and restore balance between the microbes in your body and heal any damage to tissue that occurred as a result of the infection. If you have surgery to remove a tumor, your body has to heal the affected organ(s) and knit the skin back together at the site of the incision. If you get a bone set to heal a fracture, your body has to create new bone at the site of the break.

Although Eastern, holistic, and alternative methods differ in approach, it's just as true that they are designed to aid your body's natural process of healing. You might take ginger and turmeric instead of ibuprofen to reduce the inflammation in that sprained ankle, but your body still has to regenerate the cells to heal that tissue. You may receive acupuncture to rebalance energies in your body, take supplements to boost your immune system, or receive Reiki after surgery, and they all may help your healing—that is, they will aid your body as it carries out the healing on a cellular level.

Your body is a wondrous healing machine. It is regenerative and reparative. When we are ill or injured, we have many methods we can turn to for aid. Since our body and energy body are so entwined, what can we do on an energetic level to aid our physical body in this process? This is the purpose of Healing Rays. It helps you draw upon the regenerative aspect of your sacral chakra and the soothing aspect of your heart chakra to support your body's natural healing abilities.

Healing Rays is not energy medicine. There are many forms of energy medicine, and I encourage you to find an energy healer to complement your other medical care if you have a health issue. Notice I say "complement"; it is my belief that energy medicine, holistic treatments, and alternative medical treatments should be used in combination with conventional medicine in most cases. Of course, there are ailments that may be entirely treated through energy, holistic, or alternative means. Most of the time, you will benefit from finding the right combination of both, and Healing Rays is not meant to replace any of it.

Now that I have that disclaimer out of the way and you understand what Healing Rays is *not*, we can talk about what it *is*. For one thing, women are often particularly good at this healing tool because it draws upon our sacral and heart chakras, part of our feminine pathway. As you know, our sacral chakra, among other things, is procreative energy. It's the energy of creativity, of creation, in all its forms, including the reproductive energy that creates and nurtures life. In this aspect it is the energy linked to new cell creation, cellular regeneration, and cellular repair. It is through these cellular functions that new skin cells are regenerated to heal a cut, a bone fracture is reknit, or damaged tissue is repaired.

The heart chakra is our balance point and generates an energy that helps pull all aspects of our mind and body back into balance. Many illnesses are caused by an imbalance within our system, an imbalance between the microbes in our body, our hormones, our endocrines, or our digestive enzymes. Healing is very often about returning balance to our system. The heart chakra is also our center of nurturing, soothing, and calming energy. These energies support our ability to heal by reducing our stress levels, as a high amount of stress hormones can inhibit healing.

With Healing Rays, we are combining the regenerative energies of our sacral chakra with the balancing, soothing, and nurturing energies of our heart chakra. To some extent, many of us do this instinctively when we are sick. If you get a cold and you cocoon yourself with some warm soup, your favorite book, and a bath, you are creating a nest-like energy that allows you to go inward and supports your healing process. You may be naturally bringing forth your sacral and heart energies in this case (and this is a memory you can use to bring forth these energies again in the activation steps).

With Healing Rays, we are doing this in a more deliberate fashion and are adding the palm chakras to direct healing more specifically. Located in the palms of both hands, these chakras are part of the larger secondary chakra network in various chakra systems. The palm chakras are another energy center that appears in many mappings around the world and is linked with healing. Reiki, faith healing, and Healing Touch are all examples of healing modalities that draw upon the palm centers. In Healing Rays, we will use the palm chakras to direct the energies you generate in your sacral and heart to the part of your body most in need of healing. You may not need or wish to do this, in which case you can simply generate the sacral and heart healing energies without directing them and allow them to fill your entire body.

Besides using Healing Rays to support physical healing, you can also use it to support emotional healing, by noticing where you feel a particular challenging emotion such as anger, fear, or shame in your body. We will talk more about this in the Using Healing Rays section of this chapter. Of course just as Healing Rays is meant to augment, not replace, physical medical care, it also is meant to augment, not replace, mental health care or counseling. Healing Rays is also not meant to be a healing Empowerment for you to use on others—like all the Empowerments in this book, it is designed to empower you in your everyday life and growth. Using it is part of reclaiming the vast reserves of natural powers and energetic abilities you have at your disposal.

Linda had just found out she was facing two knee surgeries, one at a time, with months of physical therapy in between and after. Because of a heart condition, she was going to be in the hospital and a rehab facility for much of each time. While she had done a lot of research and decided this was her best option in terms of future mobility, she was dreading all the hospital and rehab center time; in past stays, she had found the environments incredibly inhospitable to actual healing. The noise, the décor, the constant disruptions—she found it all the antithesis of nurturing.

Linda was also worried about the pace of her healing. She wanted to know how she could support her healing energetically. We talked a lot about methods Linda could use to make her hospital and rehab rooms more conducive to healing, including bringing her own music, bedding, and comfort items from home. We also talked about meditations to manage her stress, and alternative means, such as essential oils, she could use to support her healing while there. But energetically, we focused on helping Linda really activate her Healing Rays so that she could feel as if she could generate this energy even when her environment was not necessarily conducive to it.

Linda was able to practice Healing Rays daily at home for three weeks before her first surgery. At home she practiced it in her ultimate nurturing space, one she had created for this purpose, filled with items she found balancing, soothing, and relaxing. She drew upon memories of times in nature when she had felt the soothing and balancing aspects of her chakras activate on their own.

As soon as she was able in postsurgery, Linda practiced Healing Rays directed at her knee, and tried to do so at least twice a day. Throughout her day she would also activate Healing Ray energy and simply rest in it for a while, without directing any into her knee, in order to soothe and balance herself. Linda had other Chakra Empowerments we had worked with to prepare her, and she switched between them as needed. For example, she used the Root Bowl to quell her anxiety presurgery, the Throat Matrix to affirm her assertiveness when talking with her doctor, and the Navel Fire when she needed to draw upon her determination in physical therapy.

Above all, Healing Rays was the energy Linda sought to connect with the most, and she felt it became a default state for her over the length of her healing process. She came through both surgeries and rehab with flying colors and regained full mobility. She believed all her energetic Empowerments had helped her, and that spending so much time with Healing Rays in particular had changed her energy for good. She found she could draw upon it quickly, as soon as she began to feel stressed or a minor headache or stomachache come on, and reverse the discomfort almost immediately.

Linda's story demonstrates how you might make use of multiple Empowerments in a given situation. Of course you can't always do the entire activation process, and you won't need to once you've taken the time to cultivate your familiarity with each Empowerment at home. The most important aspect in each case is the feeling; in Linda's case, she took special care to cultivate this feeling by creating a custom space in her home in which to practice Healing Rays. In the end, this ended up being much more than a healing aid for her— it opened her up to an entirely new way of being in her body.

Activation Steps

Because this Empowerment draws upon your nurturing and comforting energies, it is helpful to practice it in a very nurturing, comforting environment. Sit in an area of your home that is particularly "yours." Perhaps light candles, incense, or bring flowers into this space—whatever helps you feel safe and nested. Wrap yourself in your favorite blanket or sit in your favorite chair. Once you have become adept at generating the Healing Rays, you will be able to do it anywhere, and it often may be when you are in places that feel the opposite of nurturing to you, as in Linda's case.

You may also want to remind yourself of your Sacral Lotus and Heart Star When You Have Felt This Before memories. Focus in particular on memories of the regenerative or reparative energies of your sacral center, and the soothing and nurturing energies of your heart. These memories may be useful to you in terms of generating the energies needed for Healing Rays.

Note that if you are simply trying to soothe yourself, you can skip steps 5 through 7, and sit in step 4 for as long as you like. If you would like to specifically direct Healing Rays into parts of your body, continue with all steps.

Step 1: Sit comfortably, take note of your nurturing surroundings, and take a few deep breaths to center yourself.

Step 2: In the location of your sacral chakra, instead of a lotus, visualize a beautiful sunset-colored, open rose. This rose has radiations of pink, yellow, and a coral orange light. Sit for a while and feel this beautiful, delicate rose and these sunset-like rays in your sacral center.

Step 3: Imagine these pink, yellow, and coral rays of light are emanating up to your heart chakra, where they create another rose made of light of the same colors. Visualize this beautiful rose in your heart center. See and feel the gentle yet powerful connection between these two centers.

Step 4: Cultivate a feeling of the regenerative and reparative energies of your sacral and the soothing and nurturing energies of your heart. Use memories from When You Have Felt This Before if you like. Take the time to generate the feeling of these two chakras specifically generating these particular energies.

Just sitting like this is healing in and of itself. Drawing these two centers together can create tremendous feelings of bliss and well-being. If you like, you can stop right here and just imagine this light filling your whole body for as long as you like. You can take a mental snapshot of this feeling to draw upon quickly at another time and continue with the affirmations in step 8.

Step 5: If you are going to move on to direct this light, visualize these rays of pink, yellow, and coral light radiating out from your heart into each arm, down into the palms of your hands. Take a moment to visualize and feel rays of yellow, pink, and coral light swirling off of your palms. If you like, you can hold your palms just a couple inches apart from each other, and imagine you're holding a ball of light of this color. Be sure to maintain the visual and sense that this energy is sourced from both your sacral and heart. Sometimes imagining holding this ball of light will help you to really connect to the light emanating from your sacral and heart into and out of your hands.

Step 6: Hold your hands, one or both, in front of the part of your body to which you would like to direct this healing light. For example, if you have a headache, hold your hands an inch or two in front of or above where your head hurts. If you have a stuffy nose, hold your hands in front of your nose or over your sinus passages. If you have a stomach-ache, hold your hands in front of where your stomach hurts the most. If you are working to aid healing of an injury that does not hurt at the moment (e.g., a damaged joint) direct the rays to wherever the pain is most prominent when you do feel it. If you are working on an emotional wound (covered in the next section), hold your hands over the spot where you most feel the emotion involved.

Step 7: Imagine the yellow, pink, and coral rays of light flowing from your sacral and heart, down your arms, out your palms, and into the area you are focused upon. The supply of this energy is limitless, sourced from the inner core of your sacral and heart chakras, so this outpouring does not drain you. On the contrary, you feel nurtured, soothed, and blissful. Sit with this visual and feeling for as long as you like.

Step 8: When you are ready to stop directing rays, imagine the light flowing down your arms into your palms has ceased, leaving only the sacral and heart roses connected. Take a mental snapshot of your feelings. Then affirm your self-healing capabilities:

> I am self-healing.
> I soothe, nurture, and care for myself.
> My capacity to heal is unlimited.
> I rest in bliss and self-love.

Step 9: When you are done, dissolve the light from your palms back into your heart, then from your heart back into your sacral, and just sit in silence and comfort for a period of time.

Using the Healing Rays

The easiest way to use the Healing Rays is for minor everyday maladies, by directing the Rays into the part of your body that is experiencing discomfort. So if you have a headache, stomachache, sore throat, or sore muscle, hold your hands right in front of the source of pain in each case. Be sure to take the time to fully generate the sacral and heart visuals and energies first, before directing the Rays through your hands. As always, once you have become proficient at this, you will be able to call upon the Empowerment quickly with your snapshot memory.

If you have a viral or bacterial infection—for example, a cold or stomach bug—there are two different ways you might work with the Healing Rays. You can direct Rays into the area of most discomfort—a stuffy nose or distressed colon—or you can sit instead in step 4, steeping yourself in balancing and nurturing energies in order to aid your body's ability to restore its internal balance.

The Healing Rays can also be used in conjunction with the Root Bowl to boost your immune system, since the root chakra is linked to our immunity. For this purpose, you would first activate the Root Bowl, and then activate the Healing Rays and rest in the energies of step 4. You may want to combine Healing Rays with other Empowerments, to the extent that you feel your malady has an emotional or mental component. For example, if it is stress related, you may also use the Root Bowl; if you've become sick after a breakup, perhaps you need some Heart Star; if you have a headache and feel frenetic, maybe you need the Navel Fire. The combinations are endless, and the point of the Chakra Empowerments is that you intuitively know what you need much of the time and can give it to yourself.

Consider now the mind-body connection and emotional healing. Many maladies do have an emotional component, and since our energy body provides a link between our physical and emotional selves, all of the Chakra Empowerments can also be physical healing aids. Many women find that physical maladies that have plagued them for years will begin to dissipate when they work long term with a chakra to heal a deeper issue. You can also use Healing Rays in conjunction with another Empowerment as part of an ongoing emotional healing process.

To do this, you will need to develop your somatic awareness—your awareness of where you feel particular emotions in your body. Specifically, the emotions you are working through—for example, you may be working long term with the Root Bowl for anxiety, with the Sacral Lotus for shame, with the Navel Fire for anger, or with the Heart Star for unworthiness. Although these emotions are linked to the chakras associated in terms of energetic blocks, you do not necessarily feel those emotions in the part of your physical body near that chakra. You may experience anxiety as butterflies in your stomach, anger as a tension in your jaw, shame as a cringing in your gut, or unworthiness as a gulping in your throat.

You may also experience these emotions energetically—perhaps you feel anger as a lump of black, thick fog in your throat or shame as a hard, green ball in your chest. Somatic sensations and awareness are very individual. It may take you some time to tune in to this, especially if you have any patterns of disassociating from your body. Many healing modalities focus specifically on somatic awareness as a starting point; if this resonates, I encourage you to look into them (and if you do feel you have tendencies to disassociate, somatic work will especially benefit you).

To work with Healing Rays in this way, take a moment to recall a related memory—a situation in which you felt the emotion you would like to work with. Do not relive the entire memory, just recall enough to trigger the emotion. Then tune in to where you feel the related energy the most within your body. Activate Healing Rays, and direct it through your hands into this part of your body. If you are combining your work with work on another Chakra Empowerment, do the somatic recall first, then Healing Rays, and then activate the Chakra Empowerment you feel is most directly related to the emotional pattern you are working with.

Regardless of how you are working with Healing Rays, it's important not to blame yourself for being sick or not healing as well as you would like. Self-blame is often a harmful side effect of pursuing mind-body help. If you start thinking "I must not have meditated enough, or eaten enough organic foods, or taken the right supplements," you've fallen into this trap. Life and the forces behind it are bigger than our understanding, and no healing system is able to account for it all. Although we can't control every aspect of our health, there is a lot we can do to increase our wellness, slow and ease our aging, and decrease our chances of becoming seriously ill. Using Healing Rays may be one piece of this puzzle for you.

Women's Energetics: Self-Care

As already mentioned, Healing Rays can be a particularly helpful Empowerment for women, because it draws upon our sacral and heart chakras, although if you have blocks to those two chakras, it may be difficult for you to access this energy. In that case Healing Rays can actually be a companion Empowerment for helping you bring forth these energies as you also work with the Sacral Lotus and the Heart Star (just as the Second Skin can be helpful when working with the Root Bowl and Navel Fire). On the other hand, if Healing Rays comes easily to you, you may want to explore training in other energy healing modalities.

For many women, Healing Rays becomes a go-to self-soothing and self-care Empowerment. If you have the habit of running yourself ragged and putting everyone else first, working with Healing Rays will provide some much-needed rejuvenating me-time (and of course, work with those patterns through other Empowerments too!). Just the act of activating these energies is healing and self-nurturing, even if you don't direct them.

Although I advise against using Healing Rays on other people, the one exception is if you are mother to or a caretaker of a baby or young children. The Healing Rays energy is a variation of the heart and sacral energy we instinctively generate toward young children when we are bonding or holding them in our lap. When they have a stomachache or headache, you can direct Healing Rays into their body (of course, never as a replacement for medical care). The primary reason I do not advise using Healing Rays on others is that it is complicated to direct healing energy into someone without taking on their energy. As our children gain energetic independence from us, they will fall into this category too. As a precaution, unless you feel you are very well-boundaried or perhaps have received training in other healing modalities, keep Healing Rays for your own self-care.

Due to its link to our feminine pathway, Healing Rays can be an especially effective complement to medical treatments for reproductive related issues including ovarian cysts, uterine fibroids, endometriosis, and pregnancy loss.

Nima had been sexually assaulted as a teenager, and again in her twenties. Although she never spoke of her attack in high school, she reported her later assault, but her assaulter had never been charged. The investigation process had been exhausting and demeaning, and although Nima had received some counseling, she eventually sought to put the entire devastating experience behind her and focus on her graduate studies.

Now at twenty-nine, Nima had completed graduate school and was a research assistant in a social policy institute. She was very focused on her career and did not date or socialize much outside of the occasional work event. But even without sexual activity, she had begun experiencing regular urinary tract infections and had had an ovarian cyst removed two years earlier. She was on and off antibiotics for the infections and had just found out she had a new cyst. She was researching alternative means of preventing both and wanted to include energetic work. Nima had read about the sacral chakra and knew that in energy medicine, both the bladder and ovaries were linked to it in women. She felt that her own sexual trauma was being held in her body in this area, leading to the recurrence of her UTIs and cysts.

We began with Sacral Lotus work and other related work to support the release of trauma from this part of Nima's body, as well as to heal lingering feelings of self-blame and anger. We also activated the Healing Rays, and I guided Nima in directing the healing energy to both her urinary tract and her cyst, visualizing the cyst dissolving as she did so. I recommended Nima activate the Sacral Lotus daily at home followed by using Healing Rays in this way.

Nima had many experiences as she worked with the Sacral Lotus on her own. She realized she had entirely suppressed her sexual energy after the second assault and was still harboring many challenging emotions. As she continued to work with the Healing Rays, she started to direct some of them to where she felt these emotions as well. As she became more comfortable with the Sacral Lotus, she also became more adept at feeling the energy of the Healing Rays. She began to use it regularly to soothe and balance herself throughout her day, in addition to continuing to direct it toward her urinary tract and cyst.

With time, Nima's cyst dissolved and she stopped experiencing UTIs. She was using other healing methods as well, so there is no way of knowing which was more important in her healing process. However, the Sacral Lotus and Healing Ray work helped Nima feel as though she had gained much more than physical healing. With the Sacral Lotus, she reclaimed her sexuality as a positive aspect of herself, and with the Healing Rays she learned how to self-soothe and balance. Developing somatic awareness was also very useful; it helped Nima recognize ways she had been disassociating from her body by escaping into her mind through her studies.

Each chakra is linked to various organs and glands in our physical body, so working to heal emotional issues associated with a chakra will often aid healing in those organs and glands as well. Energetic work should never be the only form of treatment; as in Nima's case, it may offer additional benefits. This can be especially relevant for sexual trauma survivors—trauma and related emotions are held in the body, and energy work can be a valuable part of helping to release them.

Sexual Trauma Healing: Somatic Awareness

The Healing Rays can be of benefit to you in a variety of ways as you work to heal from sexual trauma. Experimenting with it is part of a larger process of owning your own power and believing in your capacity to self-heal. As in Nima's case, you may believe you have physical maladies that are magnified or even caused by your experience of trauma; in that case, working with Healing Rays along with other Chakra Empowerments can be a valuable part of your healing.

For many survivors, the most benefit comes from tuning in to emotional somatic awareness. If you have any tendency to disassociate from your body, identifying where you feel emotions in your body and sending healing energy there, can be life changing. The emotional recall and identification process bring you into a different relationship with your body, in and of itself a potential part of your healing. If you particularly resonate with this use of Healing Rays, you may want to consider other somatic healing methods— I have included information on some on the book website.

ELEVEN
Feminine Pathway: Your Sacred Power

Related Chakras: All seven, but the second/sacral, fourth/heart, and sixth/third eye are emphasized

Energies: Flow, energy movement and connection, change, transition, wholeness, feminine power and aspects, manifesting

Use For: Life transitions, manifesting ideas, balance between chakras, postmenstruation, fertility support, postpartum, perimenopause, post pregnancy loss, posthysterectomy, precursor to sex, or anytime to connect with feminine power

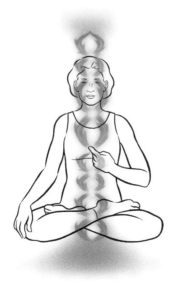

Your feminine energy is exquisite and powerful. When it is fully activated, your inner beauty is fully on display. As women we are bombarded by outlandish ideas of beauty, all physically based. The kind of beauty I am talking about is a glow, a dynamism, a centeredness, and perhaps a charisma that emanates from a woman when she is in her feminine power. It is indefinable, and yet you know it—and are likely drawn to it—when you see it. It has nothing to do with whether a woman has symmetrical cheekbones, a wrinkle-free forehead, toned abs, or even a bright aura (although feminine power certainly shines through our aura). Her Feminine Pathway is alight, plain and simple.

These last two Chakra Empowerments, Feminine Pathway and Rainbow Abundance, are culminating Empowerments in that they both utilize all seven chakras we have been working with. However, Feminine Pathway is the culmination of Women's Energetics Empowerment because it focuses primarily on the flow between our feminine, or yin, pathway chakras—the second/sacral, fourth/heart, and sixth/third eye. It differs from the other Empowerments in that it isn't designed to be used on the spot or as needed. Instead, it is an Empowerment designed to support you during particular phases of your life—transitional periods and/or when you are working to manifest an idea. To use it in these ways, you will activate it daily for a few days, a few weeks, or a few months, depending on the phase.

The Feminine Pathway differs in other ways. Because it is based in Women's Energetics, it is particularly useful during reproductive-related transitions—those tied to our cycles and phases. It also has an upward and downward version. You will build the visual you see in the image one infinity symbol (∞) or figure 8 at a time—from the bottom up to empower your *upward* pathway, and from the top down to empower your *downward* pathway.

The upward pathway is associated with personal growth and spiritual development. Many spiritual traditions with practices based on the chakras focus on bringing the kundalini energy up from the root chakra to the crown to facilitate spiritual realization. This Empowerment is not specifically designed for that, although it does trigger this upward flow as it relates to personal change and shifting into a new "version" of yourself. Whenever we undergo big transitions in our life—a new job, marriage, a new child, divorce, a move—we are called upon to adjust. We can dig our feet in and resist, or we can go with the flow and grow as a result. Often as we adjust, we will be asked to develop new skills or call upon parts of ourselves we hadn't been aware of before. In a sense, we "upgrade" almost like an upgraded software version of ourselves.

At other times we feel as if we are actually going backward. Facing divorce, illness, or job loss certainly doesn't feel like an upgrade. And for your day-to-day life, it may not be. Inwardly, any situation can foster personal insight, the development of new wisdom, the discovery of new resources within yourself, and more. It can become an inward turning point. In this sense the upward variation of the Feminine Pathway can help support you in whatever type of transition you are experiencing—one you have chosen and are looking forward to, or one you have not and are suffering through.

While the upward Feminine Pathway is about transition, the downward version is about manifesting—specifically, the kind of manifesting we do when we seek to make an idea we have into reality. Think of planting a sapling—you create a hole in the earth, plant the roots, and support them with water until they take root. Whether your idea is for a business, a product, a book, a home, an event, or something more abstract, it starts in your head (or becomes conscious there) and needs to be brought down into reality, the earth. The downward Feminine Pathway supports you when you are in a phase of your life in which you are manifesting in this way.

Thus far, our focus has been on single-Chakra Empowerments, or in the case of the Second Skin and Healing Rays, two-Chakra Empowerments. But the flow and balance *between* chakras is just as important. If one chakra is overdeveloped and another underdeveloped, or if you have blocks in one that keep energy from flowing, it affects the entire flow—in other words, it has an impact on both your ability to bring about and process change (upward flow), and your ability to manifest an idea (downward flow). Something gets stuck. The Feminine Pathway is designed to help you get unstuck—to get your energy moving.

The Feminine Pathway also helps with stabilizing and balancing the flow between your chakras when they have been triggered into lots of movement on their own. This happens when we are thrust into sudden change and are forced to adapt quickly. Of course sometimes what you need in this case is the Root Bowl to stabilize (especially if you have experienced trauma), but if you feel instead as if you need to catch up to what is happening rather than ground, the Feminine Pathway can be more helpful. Sometimes, too, such changes may trigger energetic instability—erratic bursts of energy in our energy body—and in this case the Feminine Pathway can help to smooth them. Perimenopause is an example of a time in our life when bursts like this can occur spontaneously, and the Feminine Pathway can help to stabilize us.

Alicia was in her early forties and had just completed treatment for cancer, including surgery to remove her uterus, cervix, ovaries, and fallopian tubes. Her prognosis was good, but she was struggling with the feeling that she had lost part of what defined her as a woman. She and her longtime partner Tracy had never wanted children, so she did not have regrets about losing that capability. Still, some part of her felt an essential piece of herself had been lost. She also had been plunged into menopause quickly as a result of her surgery, and although she was on hormonal treatments, she was experiencing mood swings, night sweats, and difficulty sleeping. In addition, Alicia really wanted to change careers. She felt the stress of her job as a sales rep for a pharmaceutical firm had contributed to her cancer, and she wanted to shift to something less stressful and that she felt more passionate about, but she wasn't sure what.

A yoga practitioner, Alicia was also familiar with the chakras and in fact had done prior chakra work. She thought maybe losing her uterus and ovaries had affected her connection to her sacral chakra and wanted to work there. I suggested we work with the Feminine Pathway, since it addressed several energetic needs of Alicia's at once: empowering her sacral chakra as she wanted and also empowering her entire Feminine Pathway, helping her connect with her sense of her feminine power again. In addition, it would support her desire for change in her career and smooth the tumult of her sudden transit into menopause. Alicia agreed to try the Feminine Pathway daily for two weeks.

Doing so had a big impact on Alicia. On the physical level, she began to sleep much better. Something else unexpected happened, too—Alicia felt drawn to doing ceramics again, something she used to do regularly as a hobby but gave up due to time constraints. She had rented studio space over the weekend and created a simple pot but told me she had felt calmer and happier during that time than during any other activity for months.

As we talked, Alicia decided to regularly commit to doing ceramics and perhaps take a new class. She realized that part of what was missing from her life was a creative outlet and felt that working with the Feminine Pathway had helped her reconnect to this. Ceramics was in fact one of the main ways she expressed her sacral chakra energy, and she needed to bring it forth more often.

Alicia continued with her Feminine Pathway work daily, and ceramics work weekly. To support her healing, we also worked with other Empowerments including Healing Rays and Root Bowl for anxiety. In addition, Alicia worked with her doctor and a herbalist; in time her hormones and energy body stabilized and her physical symptoms subsided. She realized she wanted to work in a hands-on healing field. She had originally gone into pharmaceutical sales as a temporary stepping stone to working in the health field but had forgotten this intention. Now she was ready to bring her life into alignment with her true desires. Alicia went back to school to become a physical therapist, and also obtained training in reiki, which she incorporated into her work with patients.

Although Alicia's menopausal symptoms were brought on suddenly by her surgery, what she was experiencing is a common occurrence during this time. Alicia thought she was feeling disconnected from her feminine power because of the loss of her uterus and ovaries, but in fact she was not in alignment with her true desires for her life. She had lost touch with both her creative and healing sides, both aspects of the sacral chakra. Her hormonal shifts had exacerbated this, as perimenopause frequently triggers energy surges that need to be smoothed out with a tool like the Feminine Pathway. Working on both flow and her feminine chakras with the Feminine Pathway helped her reawaken to her true desires and take action to bring her life into alignment with them.

Activation Steps

This walkthrough is based on the upward version of the Feminine Pathway. I've provided instructions at the end for the downward pathway, which is simply the reverse—you will start at the top and work your way downward instead of upward. You may sit or stand during this process; either way, swaying side to side along with the arm movement may be helpful.

Prep your audio file if you are using it, and study the visual before you begin. Note that it is composed of four infinity symbols/figure 8s that you will be drawing in the air with your index finger in front of your body one at a time while imagining the light flowing in this pattern inside your energy body.

> *Step 1:* If you are standing, plant your feet firmly, hip-distance apart. If you are sitting, align your spine. Take a few deep breaths and center yourself.
>
> *Step 2:* Take the index finger of your dominant hand (whichever you write with) and draw a figure eight, or an infinity symbol, in the air in front of you. Accustom yourself to this shape and motion. Sway back and forth along with the swirling motion if you like.
>
> *Step 3:* Now turn your hand around and point this finger toward the ground and your lower body. Begin to draw this infinity symbol connecting the earth with your sacral chakra. At the bottom of your "eight" you point toward the earth, perhaps even touch it if you are sitting, and at the top of your 8 you point directly at your sacral chakra, between your hip bones (you do not need to touch your body). Imagine the eight midpoint crosses at the approximate height of your root chakra. Visualize a powerful flow of red-gold light, like liquid flame, mirroring the movement of your finger inside your body, connecting your sacral chakra with the earth, and crossing at your root chakra (check the image if you are not sure what I mean).
>
> Stay with this visual for two to three minutes, or longer if you like—long enough to feel as if you have the energy flowing. If your arm gets tired, you can rest it and simply visualize the energy flow, or you can switch arms.

Step 4: When you feel ready, move your hand up and begin to draw the symbol connecting your sacral chakra and heart chakra, crossing at your navel chakra. Visualize the red-gold light flowing in this pattern inside your body, connecting your sacral with your heart through your navel. Sit with this visual and energy for two to three minutes or as long as you like.

Step 5: When you feel ready, move your hand up and draw the figure eight connecting your heart with your third eye, crossing at your throat chakra. Again, you're doing this figure eight in front of your face and chest with your finger pointed at you, and inside your body you're visualizing the red-gold light flowing in the same pattern. Stay here for two to three minutes or as long as you like (rest your arm as needed, and just do the visual, or change arms).

Step 6: Finally, move your finger up and draw the red-gold figure 8 connecting your third eye with the sky, crossing at your crown chakra. The top of your 8 points to the sky, the bottom is in your third eye, and it crosses even with your crown. See the red-gold light swirling in this way.

Step 7: Now put your arm down and try to visualize all four of these 8s/infinity symbols, all four swirling flows of red-gold liquid flame light, at once. Earth to sacral chakra crossing at your root, sacral to heart chakra crossing at your navel, heart chakra to third eye crossing at your throat, and third eye to the sky crossing at your crown. Really feel and imagine these swirls of powerful gold and red light moving inside your body in these patterns. Sway back and forth if you like, and focus on the feminine energy awakening and swirling within all of your feminine pathway centers.

Step 8: Focus on the feeling as you say each affirmation:

> My power flows freely.
> I am fluid and strong.
> I am connected to earth and sky.
> I am whole and complete.

If you like, you can add a brief visual at this point related to the adjustment you are trying to make, or the idea you are manifesting.

For example, if you are adjusting to a new job, picture yourself successful and happy in it. If you are adjusting to a new baby, picture yourself holding him or her, both of you looking happy and healthy. If you are using the downward path to manifest an idea, visualize your end goal—your idea manifested in reality.

Step 9: When you feel ready, take a snapshot memory and then let the visual dissolve. Sit and breathe quietly for a few minutes.

Downward Path: If you are using this to empower the downward path, reverse the order in which you create the connections of the chakras in your figure 8s. First connect the sky to your third eye crossing at the crown, then the third eye to heart crossing at the throat, then the heart to sacral crossing at the solar plexus, and then the sacral to the earth. Still speak the affirmations at the end when the entire pathway has been activated. If you like, you can visualize your completely manifested idea at this point if this is relevant.

If your arm gets tired during the activation, you can switch arms and focus on the visual, but don't ever visualize a static 8 or infinity symbol—the movement of the energy is important.

The Feminine Pathway generates a lot of energy. You may want to sit afterward and allow it to process for a couple of minutes before you move out into the world. You may also find that doing some stretching is helpful, or doing the Feminine Pathway right before exercise so that you can stabilize this energy physically.

Using the Feminine Pathway

If you are in a phase of your life in which you would like to use the Feminine Pathway, activate it in a private space for at least ten minutes daily. You can use it longer if you like and don't feel overwhelmed, but it is hard at first to get much flow going in less than ten minutes. Approach it like a daily meditation—at the same time and place every day, preferably first thing in the morning or as close as you can to it. If that's not realistic, it's OK, and it's fine if you miss a day—work with what fits your circumstances.

Use the upward pathway when you want to bring about change in your life or are undergoing change that you need help adjusting to. The change may be something you chose or it may not. Above all, making use of the upward pathway for this purpose will help get you unstuck in your relation-ship to this change. You will begin to see new potential in your changed cir-cumstances, glean lessons or insights, or have new ideas for how to adjust. However, it isn't a healing or emotional balancing Empowerment. If you feel as though you are in crisis or need emotional support or healing, seek sup-port for it (it may include using other relevant Chakra Empowerments), but hold off on using the Feminine Pathway until you feel emotionally stable.

If you are working toward manifesting an idea, activate with the down-ward version. There are other kinds of manifesting, of course; sometimes when we say "manifesting" we actually mean "attract": a new partner, a new job, a new opportunity. We'll talk about your chakras in relation to this kind of manifesting, attraction-manifesting, in the next chapter. The downward Feminine Pathway is the most useful for manifesting *ideas*—making some-thing you have thought of real. In this case, as I mentioned in the activation steps, you can add a visual of your end goal after the affirmations.

Sometimes it is hard to know which direction of the Feminine Pathway you want to use. If you leave your job to start your own business, you are undergoing a huge change *and* manifesting an idea. In this case, you can do the Feminine Pathway both directions if you like, five minutes upward and five minutes downward. Or you can rotate days—upward one day and down-ward the next.

You can also use the Feminine Pathway in combination with another Chakra Empowerment when you feel that one chakra is overdominating or overexpressing in your life. For example, you might feel as if you are locked into controlling navel chakra tendencies, or overtalking Throat Matrix ten-dencies—in these cases there is an imbalance between your chakras, with one dominating all of the others. For this you would use both the Empower-ment of the chakra you feel is overexpressed and the Feminine Pathway, one after the other. The single-Chakra Empowerments are not just for strength-ening a chakra, they also are for balancing it—for bringing it into its purest, highest expression. Following this up with the Feminine Pathway will help to redistribute the flow and balance between chakras.

Women's Energetics:
Working with Your Cycles and Phases

Linked to our sacral chakra, and thus our reproductive cycles, the Feminine Pathway is also a tool for change, perfect for use with our reproductive phases and cycles, which are about transition. Before menopause, our body transitions each month from ovulating to menstruating, and our sacral chakra from an outward-facing to an inward-pulling energy. Our sacral transitions during pregnancy from this regular inward/outward cycle to empowering and nourishing our womb. And postpregnancy we transition to a return to this cycle and (if relevant) energetically supporting our baby outside our body. Our body transitions to no longer having this cycle in perimenopause, and our sacral chakra becomes liberated from this cycle to express even more powerfully … if we approach this transition with that intention.

All of these transitions are perfect times to use one or both versions of the Feminine Pathway. Here is how you would do so:

- *Postmenstruation:* On the last day of your period (or your best guess), and for the two to three days after it ends, activate the upward Feminine Pathway for a few minutes each morning. This will help smooth your body's transition to its outward-facing mode and help you process and integrate your inward-facing phase. As mentioned in the Second Skin chapter, the days during our period are our most sensitive, and often our most intuitive and insightful if we can tune in to this. Using the Feminine Pathway as you emerge from these days will help you to integrate whatever emerged for you during this time.

- *Fertility:* To energetically encourage pregnancy, you can activate the downward Feminine Pathway in the days leading up to your ovulation and during it. You can also activate the Sacral Lotus during this time. What I often recommend to women who would like energetic support when trying to get pregnant is to do the Sacral Lotus for a few minutes every day all month and to add the Feminine Pathway afterward during the few days before and during ovulation.

- *Postpartum:* Use the upward Feminine Pathway whenever you can in the months after pregnancy to help you get your mojo back. As we've already discussed, there is also an energy line adjustment going on, in addition to the eventual return of your cycle. The upward Feminine Pathway will help to smooth the way for all of this adjustment. This is of course not a treatment for postpartum depression, and you should consult your doctor or midwife if you are energetically struggling beyond what you feel is your normal limit. If you are already in treatment for post-partum depression, however, the Feminine Pathway can aid your recovery. Be sure you are getting the support and engaging in the self-care you need.

- *Pregnancy Loss or Termination:* The upward Feminine Pathway is also best for this, although pay attention to your other needs at this time as well. Perhaps you also need the Sacral Lotus, Healing Rays, and/or Heart Star to help heal your body and process your emotions. Self-care and support are also critical at this time.

- *Perimenopause:* Perimenopause can last months or years. Some women experience hardly any symptoms, others experience many. Whether you will benefit most from the upward or downward Feminine Pathway partly depends upon your symptoms, and even that may change during this time. With either direction, you will benefit from the focus on flow between the chakras, because often during this time we experience energetic bursts in one chakra or another as our body transitions to an irregular cycle and eventually to not having one at all. The Feminine Pathway in either direction helps to smooth these bursts.

  The downward Feminine Pathway will be the most helpful for physical symptoms such as insomnia, increased anxiety, night sweats, restless legs, or headaches (as always, see a health care practitioner too). This is because the downward pathway culminates in the earth and thus anchors and grounds the uptick of energy and bursts that on a subtle body level are linked to these symptoms. The upward pathway is more helpful for psychological processing; if you are struggling to adjust to the idea of being in perimenopause, seeking or experiencing big changes in your life at this time (as is common), or seeking to consciously enter into this phase of your life as a "wise woman." If you are experiencing all of the above, it's fine to do both directions daily or rotate. Follow your intuition—this is partly what it means to transition into this phase of your life.

- ***Posthysterectomy (Uterine and/or Cervix Removal) or Postsalpingo-oophorectomy (Ovary/Fallopian Tube Removal):*** Posthysterectomy, consider working with the upward Feminine Pathway to affirm the continued flow of energy between your sacral chakra and the rest of your energy body. If you still have a cycle but it has become irregular, you can still work with both directions of the pathway according to the guidelines above for menstruation. If both ovaries have been removed and you are thrust into menopause quickly, you may want to work with both directions of the pathway using the guidelines from above based on any menopausal symptoms you are experiencing. Either way, you may also benefit from Sacral Lotus activation to affirm and empower your sacral chakra apart from the physical organs to which it was once linked. And don't forget Healing Rays for postsurgery healing help.

  Most importantly, remember that your sacral chakra, and your entire Feminine Pathway, are fully intact—they are not dependent upon your reproductive organs, although you may need time to reconnect in a new way to this energy as your body adjusts. Attend to your emotional needs—both the psychological and hormonal transition may take a toll that needs to be acknowledged and processed. Know that your feminine power is as potent as ever, with the potential to become even more so.

As with all the Empowerments in this book, trust your intuition. Utilizing the Empowerments isn't about picking the "perfect" one each time; it's about knowing you have multiple options and you have the power to bring forth the energy you need. It is all inside you, waiting to be unlocked. If you are not sure what Empowerment to use, go with your favorite—since *feeling* is essential to activation, if you work with your favorite, you will likely connect more deeply, and however you are accessing your energy body is better than not activating it at all. You have much more wisdom inside you than you realize; connecting with your energy body in any way will help you to bring it forth.

There is one more use of the upward Feminine Pathway you can experiment with, as a precursor to, and even during, sex. Sex is of course about much more than physical connection and orgasm—it is about an energetic intimacy, and even union. This is a whole body and whole energy-body experience, and for women, a strong Feminine Pathway can enhance these deeper aspects. We receive our partner through our sacral (regardless of the gender of your partner or your position), we join with them in love through our hearts, and we experience oneness with them through our third eyes merging. The Feminine Pathway helps activate all three. In general, use the Feminine Pathway the way you would for all of the other uses I have mentioned: daily for a period of time, and see if you experience any shifts in your lovemaking. You can also activate it right before or even during sex, although this will take practice. As you orgasm, imagine the energy flowing up your Feminine Pathway (and of course, you do not need a partner to practice orgasming in this way). Sacred sexuality is a vast subject with many different traditions and techniques, far beyond the scope of this book, but experimenting with the Feminine Pathway in this way will initiate you into the deeper aspects of sex, if you are interested in exploring them.

Lacey was energetically struggling postpartum. A trained intuitive and naturopath, she combined the two skills in her successful client practice business. She was also on a serious spiritual path and had meditated daily for years (including chakra meditation), so she was used to experiencing the rise of her kundalini as she did so. She was also used to experiencing many of her client intuitions visually as she was an adept third eye intuitive. In short, Lacey had highly developed third eye and crown chakras but was also grounded and balanced in her life, as demonstrated by her successful business and overall lifestyle.

Despite bonding well with her daughter and feeling thrilled to be a mother, Lacey felt as if her own energy body had "crashed" into her lower chakras. She described energetically feeling like a pear—her lower chakras were heavy and bloated but her upper chakras were empty. She could not focus well in meditation and was not experiencing visual intuitions. All of this was causing her great anxiety; she was now four months postpartum and worried that she wouldn't regain her skills, which would negatively affect her business and spiritual growth. She was also not the least bit interested in sex with her husband—not uncommon for women postpartum, but she had always viewed sex as a spiritual and energetic experience in addition to a physical form of intimacy, so she and her husband missed that connection.

I talked to Lacey about the new energy line she was now managing with her daughter and how adjusting to this line in her sacral would take some time, but she would be successful and her daughter's need for her energy would lessen as she grew. We worked with the Web of Light so that Lacey could begin to feel that it was OK for her to close this line when needed for her own self-care and still emanate love and nurturing from her heart toward her baby—all that was needed most of the time. I then suggested she do the Feminine Pathway daily so that she could begin to tap into her sacral and feminine energy in a new way, and to move her energy upward into her upper chakras again.

Lacey worked with both Empowerments for several weeks on her own and had many insights. The first was how often she was sending energy through her mother-child line and keeping it open, even when she did not need to, e.g., when her baby was well-cared for with her husband or her mother in the next room. She was not allowing herself to relax into her own energetic integrity, and this was adding to her feelings of being scatterbrained and fatigued. By consciously closing the line in situations like this, especially when meditating, she felt an immediate shift in her ability to focus and move her energy upward again. This realization also helped her reconnect with her husband sexually, as she realized she had felt so drained she had resisted connecting with him energetically because of it.

Lacey also began to realize that she *was* having intuitions but the way they presented themselves to her was changing—she was feeling things more in her body, not necessarily seeing them visually. Although she was not yet back to working, a friend had come over and Lacey had sensed rather than seen a dietary imbalance contributing to his health issues; she was able to suggest changes and supplements to him ... and they had worked! She began opening up to the idea that her energy body and corresponding gifts had changed—not disappeared—so she began exploring how.

Lacey returned to work when her daughter was six months old and found that she experienced both visual and bodily intuitions. In fact, with time she felt more confident in her work than ever. She was confident and happy too in her mothering and her daughter's development. Her meditations changed, and in fact became more enriching as she began to understand the idea of spiritual embodiment in a new way and to feel connected to others through her heart even more deeply.

All of our reproductive shifts trigger profound changes in our energy body, and at times they can feel overwhelming and detrimental. However, whether you are dealing with PMS, postpartum drain, perimenopause, or something else, understanding your feminine energy body and how to work with it will help you not only survive these shifts but grow and thrive because of them. Like our physical body, our energy body is profound and powerful in its cycles and phases—owning this wisdom will help you to come into your own.

Sexual Trauma Healing: Transitioning to a New Framework

In many ways, owning and empowering your Feminine Pathway is the culmination of healing from sexual abuse or assault because it is about owning your femaleness as a source of strength and a gift. If you have related to your body (and by extension your energy body) as a liability, a source of shame, or "damaged goods," the Feminine Pathway will help you release these false beliefs and the associated emotional patterns once and for all. Conversely, if you have internalized sexual objectification where you think your body is all you are and your worth is tied solely to your sexual desirability, the Feminine Pathway will help you to embrace your other levels—energetic, psychological, and spiritual.

As part of an overall energetic healing process, in most cases you will want to work with some of the other Chakra Empowerments first to help release and heal primary energetic and emotional wounds, to help you feel ready to bring all of your chakras together when working with the Feminine Pathway. Take your time. Be good and gentle with yourself. Honor your sense of pacing. For example, don't dive into using the Feminine Pathway every month in coordination with your menstruation cycle if it feels like too much—there is no need to rush or force anything. It's true for every woman—these are Empowerments for you to use as you like—but I find it's especially import-ant for sexual trauma survivors to remember the value of pacing. Use these Empowerments in a way that feels natural, healing, and safe for you—don't force yourself into a model or approach that does not work for you or feels stressful or overwhelming. There is no wrong way.

The thought or feeling of "I should be doing this another way" or "I'm not getting it right" can especially be issues for sexual trauma survivors in relation to their sex lives. Healing in relationship to sex is a very personal process that can be fraught and often requires professional counseling help. Frequently, sexual trauma survivors are caught up in a lot of "shoulds"—they think they should be having more sex, not having sex at all, or having a dif-ferent kind of sex. They believe that no matter what, their sex life is "wrong," tainted somehow by their sexual trauma. But there isn't a "should"; it is what-ever feels right for you at a particular time. This is really what owning your feminine power is about—owning your right to honor what feels good to you in a particular moment or phase of your life.

As you work out what's right for you and continue on your healing jour-ney, at some point the question may arise, "What would it mean for me to be healed?" There isn't an absolute or correct answer to this, and you don't nec-essarily have to come up with one. At some point in your journey, you will not need to focus so much on healing and will instead feel as if you are focus-ing on your life. Issues will still arise; there will still be pain, challenges, and good and bad days, but they will all no longer make you feel as though they are a reflection of your traumatic experience. Some may be, others won't. Ultimately, *you are no longer defined by it.*

The Feminine Pathway may be of help for you as you make this transition … or it may not. By this point you may have found other Empowerments or even created your own. What's most important is that you know you are capable of taking care of yourself; you know what you need. Trust that.

TWELVE
Rainbow Abundance:
Your True Colors

Related Chakras: All

Energies: Your uniqueness, your essence,
your potential, your attraction field

Use For: Generating self-love, self-appreciation, gratitude,
positivity, abundance, and attracting that which is
in alignment with your best interests

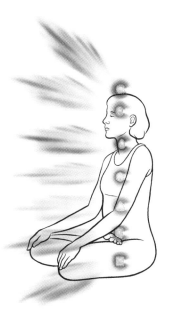

Everyone loves a rainbow. At one time I lived in an area where they were relatively common, and yet whenever one appeared, people would stop what they were doing and gaze. In the grocery store parking lot, at school pickup, or out an office window, we'd all be pointing. "Did you see the rainbow?" a total stranger might ask you in passing.

Rainbows are symbolic of good things in virtually every cultural and spiritual tradition—they represent potential, cohesion, union of earth and sky, a bridge to the future, a portal to heaven, a promise, gratitude, enlightenment, grace. Who doesn't want all that?

There's magic in rainbows, and helping you find this magic in yourself is what our final Empowerment, Rainbow Abundance, is all about. Rainbows are the sun's light reflecting off tiny droplets of water in the air, refracted at just the right angle for us to see the full spectrum of color. Each tiny droplet of water is only a part of the rainbow for a short time before it falls to the earth or joins a cloud; the rainbow appears static to us for the time it appears, but it is always in transition, always changing.

Is there any metaphor more apropos for human life? Here for a short time, our body constantly in transition, our emotions and mind ever in flux, and yet we so often think of ourselves as static, as a fixed self, the inevitable product of what has happened to us or is happening. Part of the value of working with your energy body (especially as a woman) is opening up to just how fluid and changeable we are. We are liquid light. We can grow, we can let go of an old way of being to embrace a new one, we can heal.

The Rainbow Abundance Empowerment is for resting in yourself, and allowing yourself to feel that all these energies and aspects of yourself represented by this chakra system are fully empowered, fully activated, and shining through you out into the world. You feel secure (root), inspired (sacral), powerful (navel), peaceful (heart), authentic (throat), wise (third eye), and purposeful (crown). Or you can substitute other words, other energies, from those each chakra represents. The point is that each of these is shining through you as a light, creating your own unique rainbow, and that this is the energy you vibrate out into the world.

Of course, rainbows also represent abundance … that pot of gold the leprechaun is supposedly hiding at the end. But what is abundance? Abundance is not just about money and material wealth, although those may be a part of abundance for you. But it's also about feeling rich and full physically, emotionally, spiritually. The Rainbow Abundance Empowerment is about helping you find these *within* yourself rather than focusing on getting them solely externally. This doesn't mean you shouldn't work to get what you want out in the world—many of the Chakra Empowerments can help you bring forth the energies needed to do just that. With Rainbow Abundance, you are working within a different level of yourself—you are aligning the vibration you emanate out into the world with your highest, clearest internal expression. When you do this, you open yourself up to abundance in ways you may never have conceived of on your own.

We are very prone to limiting ourselves. We are prone to thinking that if we get this one specific thing—into this school, that job, more money, this vacation, a promotion, that house, a new partner, married, divorced, a baby, this person's respect, that person's attention—we will be happy … but of course that's rarely true. At best, we get what we want and are happy for a time but eventually move on to the next want. At worst, we don't get what we want and are disappointed. With Rainbow Abundance you are taking a break from this cycle each time you activate it to just sit in the full-on energies of each of your chakras, and open to what happens.

We've talked a lot about the chakras individually and in combination as different energies, as different forces that you can bring forth. Seen from another perspective, *you as a whole* are a chakra. You are a unique doorway of energy, a unique expression of awareness in this world. There's only one of you; how energy manifests as your *particular* physical body, your particular emotions and psyche, your particular thoughts and actions—all of these comprise the way in which you express as a particular wave of energy in this vast display of energy we call our world.

Rainbow Abundance is about consciously tapping into this feeling of yourself as a unique expression of light fully empowered on every level, knowing that making yourself small serves no one. It's about your relationship to the world and what you seek to bring to it, and how you act out your desire for personal happiness. It is really about embodying all of this—*feeling* it rather than thinking it, which is what all the Chakra Empowerments are about. As you know by now, visualizing colors or saying affirmations alone isn't where the power is. It's about cultivating the feeling you want to have, or in some cases allowing the feeling to come through you. It is about *embodying* all the energies that each chakra represents.

In this sense, feeling is what is really meant when we hear about *attracting* good things into our life through our "vibrational field." There is a whole industry nowadays devoted to helping us attract money, love, opportunity, or happiness. Much of it revolves around conscious goal-setting and tools such as vision boards and affirmations to help us focus the mind and emotions on achieving these goals. Often, we are told to focus on how we will feel when we've already gotten what we want—try to feel that "as if it has already happened" feeling. Focusing on *wanting* it, this line of thinking goes, will just make us attract more lack, because the vibration we are emanating is one of *not* having, rather than having. We need to instead imagine it's already here.

This approach can be very helpful and effective, but it is often much easier said than done. Problems arise if we begin to blame ourselves when we don't achieve our goal or attract what we want. It must be our fault, we think, for focusing on wanting instead of the "as-if," or for not being positive enough, or for letting ourselves doubt too much. Once these cycles of self-blame and self-doubt begin, we can easily fall prey to feelings of unworthiness, or the belief that anything we are suffering is what we deserve.

With Rainbow Abundance, you will do something different. Instead of focusing on what you want to have or even what it will be like when you do have it, you will focus on yourself as a conduit for all the positive energies your chakras, in their most clear expressions, represent. In this way, you are putting forth your highest, most "abundant" vibration. You can combine it if you like with any other attracting or manifesting tools that you find effective, but when you put these energies forth, you are automatically emanating your highest attraction vibration. It may not be specific to a particular goal, but it is in alignment with what will benefit you and make you happy.

Through this process you open yourself up to another force—of cocreation with the universe or cocreation with God/Goddess/Spirit/Tao/Source—whatever you believe in. Instead of thinking in terms of "What do I want to create in my life?" you open to your life as an interplay between yourself and a larger force, and the idea that you can work to get what you want *and* allow in that which you might never have expected. After all, this is how we actually experience life, a back and forth between *making* things happen and reacting to things that have happened *to* us. Cocreation embraces this idea, accepting that we are not totally in control, that our life is a collaborative project with the universe, and that we need to open to new potentials we may not be able to see on our own. Our compass for this journey, our guide as we make our decisions and set our goals, comes from within.

With Rainbow Abundance, you are empowering and aligning with that inner compass by bringing forth the highest expression of every chakra all at once. You are empowering all they represent physically, emotionally, and spiritually. You are putting forth your clearest attraction vibration and opening to what comes. At the same time, you are emanating "Here I am, this is me." And though it may sound cliché, you are also saying "… and I love me."

Activation Steps

For Rainbow Abundance, you are drawing upon the image of light shining through gemstones in each of your chakras. White light is shining in your back, and as it comes through each gemstone, a rainbow is created out your front. You can think of yourself overall as a crystal, refracting white light from your back into a rainbow emanation out your front.

You will also work with words related to each chakra, preferably one per chakra. As you say these words, attempt to feel the state they represent, rather than putting them into an affirmational "I am" format. The words/ energies you choose for each chakra are up to you to select each time you use the Empowerment. You can change them as you like, and you could also use multiple words per chakra, but in general it will be easier for you to bring forth the energy if you use one per chakra.

To select these words/energies you can look back over the affirmations for the first seven single-Chakra Empowerments, or look at the following abbreviated list to get you started:

Root/First: safe, calm, grounded, resilient, stable, vital

Sacral/Second: inspired, passionate, fluid, adaptable, creative, feminine

Navel/Third: powerful, determined, centered, confident, focused

Heart/Fourth: loving, loved, balanced, worthy, peaceful, funny

Throat/Fifth: expressive, authentic, clear, honest, receptive

Third Eye/Sixth: intuitive, imaginative, insightful, wise, still, deep

Crown/Seventh: connected, faith-filled, spiritual, purposeful, meaningful

Select your word for each chakra before you begin.

Step 1: Sit as usual with an aligned spine. Take a few deep breaths to center yourself.

Step 2: Imagine there is white light pouring into the back of your body. Depending on your spiritual or religious beliefs, you can conceive of this light as God, Goddess, Spirit, Source, etcetera, or as simply energy in its raw primordial form. This light is luminous, powerful, and radiant.

Step 3: Visualize a red crystal-like gemstone at your tailbone. Imagine that this white light is coming in the back of this crystal at your tailbone, and then it's refracted out the front as a beautiful red light. This radiant red light is emanating out the front of you, even with your root chakra.

Sit with this light for a while, and then say your chosen root chakra word, with feeling and intention.

Step 4: Let the visual of your root chakra light go—we will bring all of the lights together in the end. For now, repeat this step with your sacral chakra. Visualize an orange-gold gemstone, located in your sacral chakra. See white light pouring in the back of your body through this orange-gold gemstone and radiating out the front of your pelvis as orange-gold light. Sit with this light for a while, and then say your chosen sacral chakra word with feeling and intention.

Step 5: Repeat this step for each of the remaining chakras, one at a time. In each case, see white light flowing into your back, radiating through a gemstone of the color associated with whichever chakra you are on:

Navel—yellow

Heart—green

Throat—blue

Third Eye—purple

Crown—indigo (deep blue/purple/black)

Sit with the light radiating through this chakra for a while, and then say your chosen chakra word with intention and feeling.

Step 6: Now visualize the white light radiating through all seven chakra gemstones at once. Build your visual one chakra at a time, from the root up. Then really sit with this feeling of white light pouring into the back of your body, radiating through these crystals, and emanating out the front as *your unique rainbow of light*. Sit in this for as long as you like, then dissolve the visualization and get up and go about your day.

Using Rainbow Abundance

Rainbow Abundance is like a bath of light—all of your chakras are cleansed at once, allowing them to shine forth in their full brilliance. The earlier individual Chakra Empowerments each help you focus on empowering one chakra, releasing blocks to its expression, and enabling you to use the powers it represents when you need it in your life. The multi-Chakra Empowerments also each have specific "real life" purposes—boundaries (Second Skin), energy line management (Web of Light), aiding healing (Healing Rays), and empowering the feminine (Feminine Pathway). Rainbow Abundance doesn't have a purpose in this sense; it's simply about bringing forth your brilliance. As such, you could use this Empowerment as a meditation each day, or at the end of a meditation or prayer practice if you have one. Or you could use it once a week, once a month, or whenever you feel out of sorts and a specific Chakra Empowerment doesn't seem to apply. In addition, you can use it whenever you are focused on attracting. As I mentioned in the Feminine Pathway chapter, the downward Feminine Pathway empowers the energies in us linked to bringing an idea to life. But Rainbow Abundance is more relevant when you are instead seeking to attract something into your life. It is not a specific attraction or goal-achievement tool, but you could use it with one. Activate Rainbow Abundance first, and then engage with whatever other manifestation tool you are using.

That said, attracting what we want is not straightforward. Even knowing what we want is often not simple! Rainbow Abundance involves letting go of figuring all of this out and just asking for light to come through you—for light to be expressed through you in its clearest, most colorful form. Letting go and allowing in this way opens something up in you that shifts what you attract—and often what you want—on its own.

When you don't know what Empowerment to use or are unsure of what energy you need, use Rainbow Abundance. Let go of trying to figure out your life and thinking about what you need to fix, change, or release. Just sit in your own brilliance for a time, and let that rainbow lead you from within.

In Closing: Writing Your Own Story

At this point, you may be feeling a bit overwhelmed by all the different Chakra Empowerments and unsure what to use when. If you have read all the way through this book first without working with any of the Empowerments for long, I recommend focusing on each of them for one week. As mentioned in the Introduction, you will find additional resources for helping you to do so on the book website. When that time ends, you will have some familiarity with each Empowerment that will give you the ability to use each one on the spot when a certain energy is needed in your day. Then you can contemplate which Empowerments you might benefit from working with regularly longer term.

However, trust your intuition and use these Empowerments as you see fit. There is no right or wrong way, there is only what works for you. Tapping into your energy body to any degree will change your life. It will change how you see yourself and the world. It will empower you to realize that you may not be able to control everything in any situation, but you do have control over the energy you bring to it. Through that energy, you can and do influence what happens, and how it affects you.

I have not included any usage stories in this chapter because now it is time for *you* to write your own Chakra Empowerment story. I hope the twenty-four women's stories I have offered—each an archetype for growth, empowerment, and healing—will touch and inspire you to work in this way. Even better, I hope you will choose to share your Chakra Empowerment story with me and others through the book website. There is power in sharing our stories and coming together, and I am hoping you will engage in that with me.

As I've emphasized throughout this book, we are at a turning point in history when it comes to feminine energy. We are asserting feminine power in the world like never before, throwing off old conditioning, shame, and limitations. We are redefining gender and exploring what it means to be in a female body versus a male one or a combination of both. There is a lot left to work out, and I don't claim to have all of the answers. I do believe in the importance of information and multiple viewpoints, so I hope this presentation of Women's Energetics will contribute to your own rebalancing and understanding and inspire more work in this area.

The current increase in awareness of the prevalence of sexual abuse, assault, and harassment within virtually every social structure and organization is part of the overall cultural and societal shift. The imbalances in power that have encouraged and allowed this to go on for so long are finally being challenged. Whether you are a sexual trauma survivor yourself or simply know someone who is (almost all of us do), your own healing and empowerment contribute to this shift. We are all connected energetically, and truly, one individual's shift reverberates throughout the matrix of energy and awareness of which we are all a part. This doesn't mean your own quest for healing and empowerment has to be motivated by a desire to save the world, but it can be encouraging in your darkest days to know that there is a momentum right now, that you are part of a swell. Allow yourself to tap into this larger momentum, and to be swept forward by it.

More than anything, I wish you the full spectrum of Rainbow Abundance in your life. May you be safe. May you be inspired. May you be powerful. May you be loved. May you be authentic. May you be wise. May you be filled with purpose and faith.

I honor and thank you for engaging with this book.

Please visit **www.ChakraEmpowermentForWomen.com** for additional ways to work with each Chakra Empowerment, guided recordings of each activation process, FAQ, discussion forums, and book and website listings for sexual trauma healing support resources, chakra books, and Women's Energetics information.

Index